"This book benefits practitioners and patients, wherever they may be in their journey with interstitial cystitis. Elisabeth Yaotani shares her inspirational story and provides a blueprint for healing. I recommend this book to my patients searching for a lifestyle plan to facilitate healing from within."

Dr. Cassie Jones, N.M.D.
Naturopathic medical doctor

"Even during a brief conversation with Elisabeth Yaotani I could feel her undying passion to find answers and help others like her get their life back through true healing. Throughout our partnership over the past year, her dreams for supporting those with IC and helping them achieve vitality have continued to grow, and her vast positive influence in the IC community has left me speechless.

What I respect most about Elisabeth is that she is not willing to settle. She does not cut corners, and she does not take the easy road. Instead of being complacent with the status quo, she paves her own road to health, while maintaining her integrity and values. She questions conventional methods and investigates alternative options in order to find the most effective answer, and she practices what she preaches.

Elisabeth has been where you are. She has felt every ounce of pain, the pure exhaustion day after day, and the utter defeat from every "solution" that didn't work. Hearing her story brought me to tears at one point, and my heart ached as I learned what she had gone through to get to the state of wellness she has now. Her bravery to share the intimate details of her journey in hopes of making the road for others easier is so selfless, and I am honored to work with such a genuine human being who gives herself wholeheartedly to her mission.

Elisabeth's resilient faith in God throughout her treacherous health journey is exceptionally admirable, as it would have been so easy to turn against him and blame him for her pain. Her refusal to surrender despite what seemed to be infinite roadblocks makes her a pivotal leader for all of the IC warriors who continue to battle this disease every day.

As you read this book, it's important to remember you must find your own internal motivation for changing your life, and you must be ready to change. When you believe you have no control over what happens to you, you are holding yourself back from achieving the state of optimal well-being as Elisabeth has. It is when you believe you are in charge of your health that you will see a positive change in your condition and in your life. Throughout this book, Elisabeth will light your path and give you the information you need to overcome IC, but it is up to you to apply this new-found knowledge in your own life.

Instead of focusing on how long the road might be or the effort it might take, focus on taking small steps forward. Practice self-care every single day; even the hard days. Practice makes perfect, but it doesn't mean you have to be perfect. It means you have to never give up and continue learning as you go. Perseverance has been the key to Elisabeth's success in achieving IC remission. While she cannot give you this willpower, she can inspire you with her own.

If you are feeling weary and broken down, this book will encourage you to be strong and break through any health obstacle you find yourself up against. If you are feeling lost without answers, it will inspire you to be brave and continue fighting for the state of health you know you deserve. If you are tired of suffering in pain, this book will give you hope that this does not have to be your reality any longer."

Brianne Gohlke, M.S., R.D.N.
Integrative and functional dietitian

HOW I GOT MY LIFE BACK

ELISABETH YAOTANI
WITH PATRICIA DECKERT, D.O.

MY JOURNEY WITH
INTERSTITIAL CYSTITIS

ISBN 978 1 7953 8285 4

First edition 2019

This book is not presented as an alternative to, or substitute for, the consultation of professional physicians. Instead, it serves as an additional resource, providing key information that will enable you to make an informed decision. It is always best to discuss any health-related issues with a medical professional.

References to specific corporations, organizations, products, and authorities in this book do not indicate approval by the author or publisher; nor do they indicate the approval of this book, the author or its publisher by the corporations, organizations, products, and authorities mentioned. The author is not liable for any medical outcome that may occur, whether directly or indirectly, as a result of the reader's actions in applying the methods set out in this book.

It is advised that you seek medical advice from your personal physician before engaging in any new exercise program or routine.

To my Lord and Savior, Jesus Christ,
from whom all blessings flow.

And to Tom, Alexia, Christian, and Bella.
I would not be where I am today without your
love, patience, and encouragement.
Thank you for taking care of me through this
difficult journey. You are my inspiration!

CONTENTS

ACKNOWLEDGMENTS

Rarely, if ever, does anyone accomplish significant or lasting change completely on their own. More often than not, achieving anything noteworthy requires the involvement of others. Those in our lives who have offered their support, wisdom, insights, time, and counsel deserve our gratitude and the praise that is due.

For me, this journey was fraught with tears, agonizing pain, and ongoing apathy from certain doctors, but it was also braided with hope, guidance, and, in the end, healing. I am thankful that I did not have to venture down this road alone, and that where I am today – which is nothing short of a miracle – is the result of answered prayers as well as the championing and advice of some of the most incredible people I have ever had the pleasure of knowing.

I would like to thank Marianne Rochester, M.D., who served as my urologist when I moved back to San Diego in 2008. She treated me with compassion and respect, assuring me that an answer would be found, and that I would not have to live my entire life plagued by IC. Dr. Rochester provided me with different avenues of pain management, which offered me a better quality of life. This allowed me to care for my family more effectively and to begin my journey of fitness through exercise. Her warmth and kindness strengthened me during a season in which I struggled to stay positive, and she often spoke to me at great length about my health and available treatments (as well as her interesting travels). She was the first doctor to provide me with temporary relief from my symptoms, taking excellent care of me while I was there.

A few people I knew had Donald Adema, D.O., as their doctor and praised his unconventional approach to medicine, as well as his care and concern for his patients. This made choosing him as my primary care doctor an easy decision. He was the first doctor to talk with me about testing for the methylenetetrahydrofolate reductase (MTHFR) gene mutation, and when my results came back positive for A1298C he immediately started me on methylated B12 and folate shots. He believed I would benefit from the shots and mentioned that it would help with inflammation, but I think we were both surprised at how quickly and effectively the B12 worked in reducing my IC symptoms. In addition to addressing this gene mutation, he treated me for hormone imbalance and adrenal fatigue. The results in all three areas were so impressive that I decided to share my success with others; an endeavor to which Dr. Adema lent his full support.

I wish to publicly thank Patricia Deckert, D.O., whose approach to health through the practice of integrative medicine has radically changed my life. Her expertise and guidance were directly responsible for closing the remaining gap between sending my IC into remission and restoring my health. I am not the same person I was when I first stepped into her office a couple of years ago, and I am so thankful that our paths crossed. She has the heart of a healer, coupled with knowledge and experience that brings about real change in the lives of her patients. She took this book to another level; one to which I never could have achieved alone.

I am eternally grateful to Dr. Amy Myers, who has played an enormous part in my healing process. *The Autoimmune Solution* impacted my life, providing me with information, guidance, and encouragement. I used it as a road map, and it provided me with the course of action needed to get to the root of IC so that I could deal with it head-on. I would not be where I am today had she not personally forged this path in the autoimmune community; a path she continues to light for the rest of us to follow. She is breaking down barriers and leading the research into reversing autoimmunity, for which we owe her more than she could ever know. She is a living testimony to the influence of diet and lifestyle on our health, and her dedication to helping others achieve the same success makes her one of America's leading doctors.

I am also thankful for my talented and dedicated editor Joy Tibbs, who also stepped in when needed to serve as my writer, which lifted the burden from my shoulders and helped bring my vision for this book to fruition. Additionally, I owe an enormous thank you to Brianne Gohlke, M.S., R.D., who brought her expertise to the chapter on diet by editing it as well as helping to explain the importance of "eating clean" and using food as medicine. She also contributed a number of recipes. Thank you to others who contributed recipes, especially Rose Manning.

There is one individual I need to thank for always having my back. He has been my strongest supporter through all of this. Illness can take its toll on a person, and on their loved ones. As if life and marriage were not hard enough to navigate, throwing in the additional weight of a partner who is sick can, and often does, crumble a marriage. My husband Tom stepped in and took the weight I could no longer carry on his shoulders.

He doubled down to not only financially provide for our family but to make life as normal as possible for our children, who were growing up with a mother facing significant limitations due to illness. His love, patience, and support have not gone unnoticed; and neither has the fact that he never once complained about the burden he had to carry. His love and friendship have sustained me, and I am a better person for knowing him. It was Tom's idea to write this book, and his financial support made it possible. He encouraged me to use what I knew to help others who were suffering, reminding me that if I could help just one person it would be worth it!

FOREWORD

Many of us have struggled with ill health at some time in our lives, and life can often seem unbearable for those battling chronic pain. I once struggled with serious health issues, such as my autoimmunity (visit amymd.io/mystory for further details), but have thankfully been able to overcome them. This drive to know that it is possible to recover from chronic illness is what led me to open my functional medicine practice and write both *The Autoimmune Solution* and *The Thyroid Connection*. It has long been my passion to help others achieve optimum health, and Elisabeth Yaotani shares this same commitment, as you will see from this insightful book.

Perhaps, like Yaotani, you are suffering from interstitial cystitis or some other form of chronic inflammation. Perhaps you have run with every conventional medicine your physician offered and tried every other trick in the book, but nothing seems to be working. Not only is the condition pretty agonizing; it is now affecting your ability to work, exercise, and interact with your family. Maybe you've hit rock bottom and are ready to try a different strategy.

If this description sounds familiar, you've come to the right place! This book contains page after page of wisdom from Yaotani's personal position of experience in dealing with interstitial cystitis. Through trial and error, she has uncovered ways to not only deal with the pain but to fully recover from it and get back to the lifestyle she enjoyed before her miserable journey began – perhaps even discovering a better version of herself along the way.

Yaotani delves beneath the surface to explore the root causes behind this debilitating condition and searches for ways to heal the whole body rather than focusing on the bladder in isolation. She believes a combination of "eating clean," rectifying hormone imbalance, detoxifying your body, healing leaky gut, taking the right supplements, and looking at your DNA profile to understand genetic issues are all critical elements in setting you on the path to recovery. This book contains helpful nutritional and lifestyle advice, and even provides a handy meal plan so you can get started immediately.

It is rare to stumble upon a book in which the author is candid and open about her personal experience of illness, as well as being so scientific and informative about the many methods of treatment available. If you are suffering from interstitial cystitis, you will be able to identify with Yaotani's pain and suffering, but you will also be inspired by the way she has proactively worked to reverse her symptoms and get her life back on track. There is no such thing as a quick fix or a cure for all, but by following some or all of the advice tucked between these pages you will be able to work out which steps you need to take to regain your health.

Sometimes the road to recovery involves hard work and dedication, and Yaotani makes no apologies for this. However, she is very clear about the fact that the effort you put in now will surely be worth it in the long run. The message is clear: start small, but start now! Begin thinking about the foods you eat, the chemicals you are exposed to and the medications you are taking. Consider how active you are and the way you handle stress. Think about the factors that led to you developing interstitial cystitis in the first place. And talk to a functional medicine practitioner who can support you in your journey to better health.

By making some simple but fundamental changes to your lifestyle, you may soon find that you are happier, healthier and stronger than ever. You may sleep more soundly and exercise more efficiently. You will have more energy to tackle the daily grind and to pursue your personal interests. Even your skin may be clearer! Best of all, that never-ending pain you currently feel, and the constant fear of flare-ups, should well and truly be a thing of the past. Your friends and family will notice the difference in you as you take your life back step by step.

If you're ready to start the fight against interstitial cystitis, this book is for you. And if you're not quite there yet, start reading this book anyway! Yaotani's enthusiasm will not fail to captivate and motivate you, and the lasting results she has experienced are the best possible advert for her recommended treatments. Whatever you are battling with today, I wish you all the best for a pain-free future and a longer, healthier, and happier life.

Dr. Amy Myers, M.D.
New York Times bestselling author of *The Autoimmune Solution* and *The Thyroid Connection*

INTRODUCTION

"The capacity for hope is the most significant fact of life. It provides human beings with a sense of destination and the energy to get started."

American author Norman Cousins

If you are currently living with interstitial cystitis (IC) and the debilitating pain it brings, there is hope. You can get your life back! I have been on this journey for thirteen years, struggling for a considerable portion of the way as I unearthed answers in a quest to leave no stone unturned. This book has been written as a guide to overall health and wellness through detox, gut health, diet change, and methyl genetic nutrition analysis (MGNA). Through it, you will not only learn the root causes of inflammatory illnesses, including IC, but also how to decrease your symptoms and even reverse them.

Since you are reading this book, I will assume that you or someone you care about is currently suffering from interstitial cystitis. Let me take a moment to break down what I have personally learned about this debilitating condition. IC, or painful bladder syndrome (PBS), is a bladder disorder that is characterized by chronic bladder pain, bladder pressure, bladder spasms, discomfort, lower back pain, pain in the abdomen, pain as the bladder fills, the frequent need to urinate (some report urinating upwards of forty to sixty times a day) but with little voidance, pelvic pain, and Hunner's ulcers (which affect five percent of IC patients), with symptoms lasting longer than six months. IC sufferers often experience increased pain during exercise, in seasons of stress, and even while carrying out routine activities. They may also suffer with pain during and or after intercourse, including pain in the urethra as well as the vulva and/or vagina (women), or the penis, scrotum, and/or testicles (men).

IC pain can range from dull to sharp, and may be either chronic or sporadic, with extreme bouts of pain (flare-ups) lasting anywhere from a few hours to upwards of ten days or more. Due to damage in the bladder lining, bladder scarring is not uncommon with IC. This can lead to stiffening and shrinkage of the bladder, which decreases its ability to store normal amounts of urine. Poor diet, hormone imbalance, stress, anxiety, infections, and physical activity can all trigger or worsen IC symptoms.

IC affects the lives of millions but is most common in women, with an average onset age of forty. Those with IC often suffer from other conditions, including irritable bowel syndrome (IBS), small intestinal bacterial overgrowth (SIBO), fibromyalgia, ulcerative colitis, celiac disease, chronic fatigue syndrome (CFS), prostatitis, Sjögren's syndrome, and vulvodynia. The exact reasoning behind their association is multifaceted, and conventional medicine has struggled to explain the correlation.

The exact cause of IC is still unknown, but may include physical trauma to the bladder, a genetic predisposition, allergies, recurrent urinary tract infections (UTIs), food allergies and/or sensitivity, sensitivity to certain environmental factors, intestinal permeability, neurological damage, hyperthyroidism, adrenal dysfunction, infectious microorganisms, neurogenic inflammation, pelvic floor dysfunction (PFD), toxicity, liver dysfunction, and bladder mastocytosis.

It is likely that multiple underlying factors are at work in creating what may be the 'perfect storm', given that the human body is complex and internally integrated. This makes IC a difficult condition to treat when viewing bladder dysfunction in isolation. Some medical professionals have acknowledged – and I agree – that the syndrome may be an autoimmune condition, given that the bladder wall can be primarily infiltrated by T lymphocytes and mast cells, and that many patients with IC present autoantibodies and systemic diseases commonly associated with IC. Unfortunately, there is no documented cure for interstitial cystitis at present, and in many cases it is recognized as a disability in that it can greatly affect quality of life.

Our kidneys filter our blood, collecting waste products while making urine, which runs down the ureters into the bladder, where it is stored until it is ready to be expelled from the body. Urine contains more than 3,000 chemical compounds. Seventy-two are made by bacteria, while 1,453 come from the body itself. A further 2,282 come from diet, drugs (over-the-counter, prescription, or recreational), cosmetics, and environmental exposure. The sheer volume of toxins currently lurking in the urine cannot possibly be beneficial to the bladder, as these most certainly threaten the balance of the bladder's microbiome.

A healthy bladder contains a protective layer of mucous called glycosaminoglycan (GAG), which acts as a barrier between the urine and the bladder wall. Those who suffer from IC have a defect in this protective layer, resulting in tears to the bladder lining, causing the interstitial tissues to be exposed. This allows any toxic substances present in our urine to penetrate the bladder wall, resulting in inflammation of the bladder. The bladder lining (GAG) often fails to repair itself for a number of reasons.

I have come to understand a great deal about IC and agree with those who support the position that, along with other inflammatory illnesses, it is caused by an imbalance in the body. In order to minimize symptoms and reverse this syndrome, as well as preventing other autoimmune conditions, we must consider the body as a whole and address the root causes of inflammation. In the pages that follow, I will explore ways of identifying the triggers that cause inflammation and explain the importance of removing them. I will look at: ways of detoxing the body; how to heal leaky gut; the healing power of food; using high-quality supplements to address genetic variants that are affecting natural pathways in the body; and making lifestyle changes that will reduce the toxic burden, bringing about healing and an improved quality of life.

Everything you need to effect change in your body is contained in these pages, but healing will not come about without an intentional approach. I am confident that if you make the decision to change course and do the necessary work you can get your life back, as I have. I do not have a single "cure-all pill", but I promise you that reducing and minimizing your symptoms is possible, as is sending your IC into remission. Best of all, it can be done relatively quickly if you set your mind to it.

I am an extremely private person, and I usually hold my personal life tightly in the clutches of my own hands, which has made writing this book extremely difficult. During the first couple of years living with IC I felt embarrassed and was not inclined to discuss it with others. The few people who knew about it would often ask me how I was feeling, and though I knew it came from a place of love and concern I dreaded the prying questions and would quickly change the subject. However, when I began to take my health back I became burdened for those who were suffering in the darkness of their own lives. I began to read blogs and posts from people who had shared their stories of pain and hardship in dealing with this condition, and I knew that I could no longer hide behind the curtain of self-preservation; not when I possessed knowledge that could benefit many who were desperate for help.

When I was first diagnosed there wasn't as much in the way of support or information as there is today. This guide is for those who have tried conventional medicine or antibiotics to kill off specific strains of bacteria, or even plant-based diets, only to be left feeling disappointed and empty-handed. A refusal to accept that, "It is what it is, so suck it up," fueled a personal quest that unveiled some interesting answers. When applied, these answers brought me quick results.

The first part of this book covers the story of my personal journey with IC. The second part will provide you with a guide to bladder wellness and an understanding of what is happening in your body. The most important fact I can share is the simple truth that you are not alone! You do not have to accept that struggling with IC is your lot in life; nor are you destined to live out the rest of your days with all the pain and limitations this condition can bring. It is my desire to bring hope to those who are suffering. I want to encourage you to get up and fight to take control of your health. I pray that you will be encouraged and inspired to join me in this fight against interstitial cystitis.

ABOUT THE AUTHORS

Elisabeth Yaotani
Elisabeth Yaotani is the founder of IC Wellness, an online resource dedicated to helping others in their fight against chronic pain and illness. Additionally, she writes informative articles on a broad range of health-related subjects and has developed a number of popular recipes with a focus on "eating clean" in order to bring health back to the liver, immune system, and whole body.

After being diagnosed with an autoimmune condition at the age of twenty-nine, Elisabeth realized she needed to make significant dietary and lifestyle changes in order to address the root cause of her illness and end her suffering. Having conquered debilitating pain and exhaustion, she has become a source of hope and inspiration for many others who are suffering from interstitial cystitis and other chronic conditions. Elisabeth wrote this book to inspire those who are still battling to take action and get their lives back!

Dr. Patricia Deckert
Dr. Patricia Deckert graduated from Michigan State University with the intention of becoming a science teacher. She soon became disillusioned with teaching and began exploring her real passion, medicine. She applied to medical school at age thirty-nine and graduated in 1991. Dr. Deckert studied osteopathic medicine, which teaches that physicians can help facilitate the body's natural ability to heal itself.

In 2001 she opened her practice, New Beginnings Health Care, and developed it into an integrative wellness center with multiple providers. Her key focus over the years has been attaining optimal health through gut health, hormonal balance, allergies, genetics, diet, and detoxification.

It was at New Beginnings that Dr. Deckert met Elisabeth Yaotani. Fascinated by Elisabeth's journey, she was thrilled to be asked to contribute to this book in the hope that it would help others suffering from chronic pain to regain their health.

PART 1

Chapter 1

KNOCKED DOWN

"Things don't go wrong and break your heart so you can become bitter and give up. They happen to break you down and build you up so you can be all that you were intended to be."

American author Charlie Jones

Life was pretty routine and fairly quiet in my twenties. At twenty- nine I was healthy and happy, with no major complaints. My husband of eleven years, Tom, with whom I have three children, had just moved our family from San Diego to Menifee, California, in order to simplify our lives and give us more quality time together. We were fresh into the first year of homeschooling, which gave us the flexibility to travel to Disneyland at the drop of a hat, or up to Big Bear during the winter to snowboard. We had settled into our quaint little neighborhood and even put a pool in our back yard. Things were going so well that we decided it was the perfect time to add to our family. Life was good!

We woke up fairly early one January morning to head up to Big Bear and spend a day on the slopes as a family. I did not feel well that morning and thought I had a urinary tract infection (UTI). This seemed strange to me, since I had just gotten over my second ever UTI a few weeks prior. I decided I could handle the discomfort and we headed up the mountain. We reached Snow Summit about an hour and forty-five minutes later, only to find that it was closed for the day. I was quietly relieved because I was feeling much worse by then. We decided to grab some food and hang out at the cabin.

As the afternoon wore on and I downed yet another glass of cranberry juice, I suddenly became aware that I was pacing the hallway. The bladder pain seemed to be getting worse and I knew something wasn't right. I called my obstetrician-gynecologist (OB-GYN) and made an appointment for the following day. By the time the sun set I had downed several more glasses of cranberry juice and was on the verge of screaming. The pain was excruciating. I'm still not sure whether I was trembling from the pain or the fear of an unknown root cause, but sleep was not forthcoming that night and I rotated between crying on the bathroom floor and pacing the hallway impatiently, waiting for the sun to rise so we could head back down the hill.

On the drive home I grabbed my phone the moment I had reception and began to research UTIs. During my research I came across some information about interstitial cystitis (IC), but I closed my eyes and willed it away. I refused to let the fear seep further into my mind.

A few days later my doctor's office called to let me know that the urine culture was negative, which meant I did not have a urinary tract infection. They advised me to see a urologist, and my heart sank. Deep down I knew it was IC; a condition that was, at that time, completely foreign to me.

About a week after my appointment with the urologist I had an appointment for a cystoscopy with hydrodistention. I was informed that this was an outpatient procedure and that it would be performed under general anesthesia. My doctor explained that he would insert a cystoscope (a thin tube with a light and small camera at the end) into my bladder through the urethra in order to examine the bladder wall. He would fill my bladder with fluid, then release the fluid a few minutes later to re-examine the bladder wall, this time for abnormalities. If IC was detected he would intentionally tear the lining of my bladder wall in the hope that it would grow back healthy. This was the beginning of a very long and painful journey.

The nurse shook me awake with force, and I blinked several times to clear my eyes and get my bearings. The moment I realized where I was the pain struck my body like a tidal wave. I took a few deep breaths and tried to calm myself. I did not want to be one of those emotionally driven, high-maintenance patients who annoyed the entire recovery room as well as the staff. The nurse returned and asked me to describe my pain level on a scale of one to ten. I gritted my teeth and replied that I was in terrible pain, so she graciously offered me a single 500 mg Vicodin (hydrocodone/paracetamol) tablet. As I waited for the medicine to take effect I stood up and began pacing the length of the bed.

At one point I realized my hands were on top of my head and I was pulling at my hair in an effort to maintain my silence. A tear slipped down my cheek as I struggled to remain composed, adamantly refusing to let those in the recovery room see me cry. I stuffed my pain and emotions down, bottling the noise that beckoned within to be released. About a half an hour later the nurse released me to my husband, who had just returned from the pharmacy with a prescribed bottle of Vicodin. I bit my lip until we were in the car, and then I let myself go. Tom was startled by my sobbing but wrapped me tightly in his loving arms. Then he opened a cold bottle of water and handed me another Vicodin.

We had a short drive home and my crying was beginning to dwindle as the Vicodin finally began to do its job. Once at home, Tom scooped me up and placed me in our bed to rest. He placed a heating pad over my abdomen and fully opened our bedroom window so I could listen to the sound of rain. Completely drugged and more comfortable, I drifted off to sleep.

*

I stared intently at the pictures of my bladder and tried to grasp all that my doctor was saying as he pointed to the multiple tears he had found in my bladder lining during the procedure. I remember feeling like I was in a dream; that this could not be happening to me.

"So what do I need to do to get better?" I asked.

It was a stupid question, since I knew there was no cure.

He responded with: "One-third of IC patients get better on their own and it simply goes away. One-third remain the same and the other third get worse over time."

He went on to say that the experts did not know the root cause of IC or how to cure it, and that they had no explanation as to why some patients got better or worse over time. He informed me that IC patients fall into three categories: mild, moderate, and severe.

The next question I asked felt like my last ray of hope. "Where am I on the scale?" I asked.

"I would put you at moderate to severe," he replied.

Hope seemed utterly and unequivocally lost at that moment, and despite having a firm policy of not crying in front of strangers I simply couldn't help it as the moisture that had filled my eyes suddenly spilled down my face. Though I felt embarrassed, the feeling of hopelessness outweighed my sense of pride. I grappled internally with the fact that my life would never be the same; that I would always be in that amount of pain; that there was no medical cure available to rid my body of this agonizing illness. Despair reared its ugly head as I hung mine in defeat.

The doctor discussed a couple medications with me that have proven to help some IC patients. Elmiron and heparin were discussed, but I placed them on the back-burner since it felt like trying these medications meant I was accepting the condition by signing on the dotted line. Then, as quickly as the despair had knocked me down, something inside me shifted as defiant rebellion filled my blood. I walked out of his office that day resolving within myself to find a cure if it was the last thing I ever did. I dug my heels in and refused to accept a life sentence.

For most of my life, stubbornness has been my Achilles heel. This time, though, I knew that it could be harnessed for good. I began researching everything I could about IC. People had plenty of suggestions, ranging from specific vitamins to antibiotics. Since I had left the doctor's office with one bottle of Vicodin and another of Pyridium (phenazopyridine), along with a long list of foods I could not eat (which seemed like just about everything), I figured I had nothing to lose by becoming a guinea pig.

I seemed to get worse in the days that followed, and it became increasingly difficult to carry out my daily activities as I was in constant pain. Walking a block became a challenge, as did caring for my family. The usual distractions during the day helped me focus on the pain a little less, but night-time was very different. I was up every twenty to thirty minutes to go to the restroom, and trying to fall asleep in the midst of the pain became my greatest challenge. It took a long while to doze off, only to be woken moments later to go to the bathroom... again. Days would pass with hardly any sleep, and the pain medication and heating pad became my nightly companions. There were days when I spent most of the day in bed, and the frustration led to me crying and sulking over my situation.

Then one day I decided to switch gears mentally and to quit feeling sorry for myself. Instead, I chose to use the time to count my blessings, one by one. Oddly enough, I began to feel a sense of hope because I believed God was doing something in me and through me by means of this illness that I didn't quite understand. I thanked Him for waking me up, for giving me life, for my three healthy children and my sweet husband; for our home, the food on our table, the birds chirping outside, the sun shining, and so on. Despite how grim my outlook seemed I knew full well that it could always be worse, and therefore I had something to be thankful for. Though my life had changed I was still blessed beyond measure, and I took the time to examine just how blessed I truly was. This had a profound effect on my day-to-day life, and the sulking came to an abrupt end.

During extreme flare-ups, two Vicodin only managed to cut the pain in half, and though I was grateful it still meant more sleepless nights. I began sleeping with the television on all night since I was up anyway, and this served as a legitimate distraction from the constant pain. Life had changed. My diet was extremely bland, and I only drank water. I avoided citrus, caffeine, spicy foods, processed foods, soy, alcohol, vitamins, and seasoning. I veered away from anything acidic as well as certain fruits, nuts, and vegetables. I could no longer play in the pool with my kids as the pool water irritated my bladder. Snowboarding requires the use of the abdomen, so our time on the slopes was significantly reduced. It hurt to stand and walk, and car rides jarred my bladder, which intensified the pain. Even something as simple as sitting in church for an hour and a half was difficult because the pain of sitting up straight while remaining still seemed to irritate my bladder further.

I felt pain if there was liquid in my bladder and pain after trying to empty it. I found myself trying to remain still – I preferred lying on my side – as much as possible to reduce irritating my bladder through movement, which consequently led to me putting on weight. When the pelvic pain was extremely severe it caused a nerve running down my right leg to act up, and over time I developed a slight limp on my right side when I walked. This made hiding the condition a little more difficult, and I became embarrassed as I didn't want my health issues to become a topic of discussion.

There were about three nights in the first year when I remember getting up to go to the restroom and the pain being so strong and sharp that the second my feet hit the floor the rest of my body followed suit. The first night I just lay there and cried until the pain had died down enough for me to crawl to the toilet. The second time it happened I spent about two minutes crying in the darkness of my room and then decided I would just spend my time on the floor in prayer. The third time it happened I began to pray immediately. I figured if I was going to be on the floor I might as well make use of the downtime and spend my time talking to God!

The most heartbreaking struggle of all was that I began to experience intense pain while being intimate with my husband. He took a temporary step back in response because he didn't want to hurt me, and as a result I began to feel isolated and alone.

When we lose our health we become limited and walled in by those limits and constraints as the simplest of tasks become enormous challenges. I remember struggling to clean the house, and one day in particular I pushed myself beyond my limits to get it all done. By the time Tom got home that evening I was curled up in a ball on the bed. He greeted me in his usual chipper way and said he wanted to go out and do something. But I knew that I was done; that I had pushed myself beyond my limits and that I simply couldn't move. I wanted to remain as still as I could for the remainder of the night.

He became upset at seeing me curled up like that, riddled with pain. He let me know that he did not want the house to be the cause of my pain, and that he would be hiring a housekeeper. I hated the thought of someone coming in and doing what I considered to be *my* job. I felt as though accepting help at that point meant I was somehow accepting that I was useless. I cried in defeat, but he gently held me and let me know that he would much rather have me up and in less pain when he got home, because that was far more important to him than a clean house. I agreed to let him bring someone in, and at the end of the day it was a huge help; not only for me, but in the best interests of our family.

As bad as things were, I learned to make a point of enjoying life on a daily basis. It's a habit I formed when my kids started school. Life can get hectic and days can be long. As parents, we have days that are less than pleasant. When we feel stressed out and worn down we may have a short fuse with our children at times. I introduced a ritual in which we would stop everything and shut the world out for thirty to sixty minutes a day. We would make popcorn or grab some fruit, chocolate, ice cream, or candy (for them, not me), then curl up on my bed or the sofa and either watch a funny show or play a game.

The only priority I had was laughter. This allowed us to connect and unwind, and on many occasions I used this time to apologize to them for my lack of patience. I love to laugh, and I make this a daily priority. I love that our home is filled with laughter, and that the sound of my children's laughter is forever engrained in my memory. The problems of life don't seem as large or feel quite as heavy when you can smile and laugh in the midst of the pain. God never promised that life would be free of difficulties, pain, and heartache; quite the opposite, actually. He did, however, promise that He would be near the broken-hearted, and an ever-present help in times of trouble. I am thankful that He is forever faithful and always present in the life of every believer. He is my constant source of hope and joy.

Chapter 2

WHERE THERE'S A WILL

"Pain is one element, but what comes from pain can shape, break, or strengthen the deepest parts of our being."

My son, Christian Yaotani

My refusal to accept the diagnosis as a permanent fact and unmitigated sentence led me on a journey of experimentation that has left me with a few regrets. My desperation, coupled with my strong-willed personality, resulted in me trying to cure my IC with an extremely high dose of antibiotics. It was the first "answer" I had uncovered in four months, and I was too focused on the end result to worry about the potential consequences that lay hidden in the shadows.

My online research had led me to someone who claimed that IC was caused by certain bacteria and could thus be cured with a high dose of antibiotics. A urine broth culture was recommended to see if this strain of bacteria was present, but at the time my doctor didn't know of any lab that offered this type of test, so I proceeded blindly. I purchased this individual's book and set aside a couple of weeks, allowing me time to rest while I focused on tackling the condition head on. My urologist at the time was hesitant to prescribe me the antibiotic Doxycycline at the level I was asking for, since it was three times the normal dose. I convinced him that I had found someone who had the backing of a medical doctor. He wrote me the prescription but warned me that such a high dose could have side effects.

Our bodies have a natural way of informing us that they do not agree with some of the unnatural things we try to put into them. Trying to ingest the high dosage of antibiotics became an extreme challenge as my body literally struggled to swallow the fifth and sixth pill each day. The book made it clear that vitamins needed to be taken daily in order to counter the damage antibiotics can have on the body. I followed each step in the book, which provided clear, in-depth instructions on how to care for one's body. The author even recommended that the sufferer's partner take the antibiotics, since the bacteria could apparently be transmitted during intercourse, which Tom dutifully did.

I subsequently completed the recommended follow-up series of antibiotics, but to no avail. Not only did the medication make absolutely no difference with regard to my IC, but my immune system was shot to pieces. Prior to the treatment I would get sick about once a year, and I would brag that I could beat almost any virus in twenty-four hours. That was not the case after completing the course of Doxycycline. In the years that followed I could feel the weakness in my system and picked up just about any virus I came into contact with. Worse still, it would take me a week or longer to get better. This inevitably resulted in a weakened and extremely vulnerable immune system.

I am not discounting the author's claim to have cured herself, nor the fact that she has helped many women over the years. What I would suggest is that IC may be caused by a number of factors, and since we do not know what they all are, a single "cure-all" solution will not work for everyone.

Let me also take a moment to say that I believe many people have been incorrectly diagnosed with IC. Many sufferers are diagnosed based on symptoms they have told their doctors about, a negative UTI test, and nothing more. Due to potential side effects, diagnostic testing by means of a cystoscopy with hydrodistention is no longer considered a preferred practice in diagnosing IC. Furthermore, medical experts are beginning to subcategorize IC, which means bacteria could be to blame. I believe everyone needs to address this issue, but whether bacteria are the root cause remains to be seen. Medical trials have shown that, despite the type or combination of antibiotics used, and the duration they were taken for, this form of treatment is not effective against IC.

One young woman I discovered on the internet began a blog about her journey with IC and the "cure" she had found. However, a red flag went up for me when she shared some of her diet tips. She acknowledged that those with IC cannot drink alcohol because it irritates the bladder, but recommended vodka and lime, which she claimed was the most tolerable alcoholic option. As an IC sufferer, let me just say that vodka and lime is one of the worst things you could put into your system. It's a recipe for disaster!

After the antibiotics failed to cure me, my doctor urged me to begin a series of heparin bladder installations. I agreed, and with little knowledge about it allowed one of his nurses to start the treatment series that very afternoon.

Let me start by saying that I love nurses – some more than others, of course – and have great respect for what they do and the dedication they bring to the job. But the nurse that afternoon was young and struggled to get the catheter in. Catheters are painful enough as it is, but add a struggle and suddenly I'm using all my restraint to keep myself from kicking this poor girl. She finally got it in place, emptied my bladder of urine and administered the heparin treatment. I was instructed to hold it for at least forty-five minutes, or as long as I possibly could.

I left the office upset and in pain, but pulled myself together and took my daughter to gymnastics. I sat in the lobby watching her practice and was relieved that the pain was finally beginning to die down. I waited forty-five minutes and then went to the restroom to empty my bladder. I was in no way prepared for the level of pain that was to hit me as I did so. Sitting in the stall shaking, I didn't know what to do next. The pain was so intense that I didn't think I would be able to drive us home. I waited ten minutes in the stall until I could compose myself, then made a dash for the car. Thankfully it was dark by then, and I shut myself in the car and sobbed. The pain was so severe that I had to call Tom at work and ask him to come home.

My daughter's class filed out a few minutes later and she hopped into the car. I drove us home in tears. There was no other option, since Tom was almost two hours away. Once home, I immediately climbed into bed. Not only was my bladder extremely irritated, but every time I moved over the next two days I felt intense pain. Whenever I needed to urinate I would postpone it for as long as I possibly could, fearing that I would bleed as a result of how cut up I felt on the inside. I did not return for my next treatment a few days later, and swore off the heparin for a year and a half.

It was at this point that I decided to give Elmiron a try. There wasn't a lot of medication on the market, and Elmiron was pretty much it as far as oral treatments went. Although I only stuck with it for a few months I saw no results during the time I was on it. My frustration began to grow, and my patience was wearing thin. During one visit I shared with my doctor the level of pain I was living with daily, along with my growing frustration.

He told me: "Some IC patients live in constant pain, leading them to have their bladders removed."

He said this was a last resort and not one he recommended, because some IC sufferers still reported having "phantom symptoms" even after their bladders were taken out. My heart sank as fear crept in. I left that day wondering if having my bladder removed altogether was the direction in which my journey would take me. The thought was too much for me, and I crumbled under the weight of my fears once again.

More than two years had passed since I was first diagnosed with IC, and unfortunately the economy had taken a turn for the worse. We decided that my husband's commute to work was taking its toll, so we headed back to San Diego. By this point I was often able to manage through the daytime without pain medication, but the nights were still terrible. I used painkillers to reduce the pain, the heating pad to soothe it so I could sleep, and the TV to distract my mind. I wasn't exercising at all; in fact, there were times when I couldn't even walk.

The first year with IC was the worst, as I also struggled with depression and anger. By the second year I was no longer angry; I was, however, far more discouraged and exhausted. During the first year I wrestled with trying to understand the meaning behind it all, questioning what I had done to deserve such a heavy and unfair burden. I fought to keep my head straight and to focus on the positives, but there were days when the pain got the better of me. There were moments when the darkness covered me like a cold, wet blanket as hopelessness engulfed me.

The times when I couldn't get the pain to quiet down to a tolerable level – when I couldn't get comfortable no matter what I tried, or sleep through the pain – were the most difficult to withstand. I felt physically trapped and utterly mastered by the illness that enslaved me. As I look back now it seems silly, but for the first year I thought God was punishing me for something terrible I had done, and I was angry. I wasn't sure what I had done exactly, but I reasoned that it must have been something awful to deserve such a terrible lot in life.

This mindset often dominates my thoughts whenever I focus my attention solely on the storm that besets me. The sheer magnitude of the storm can engulf me, and the longer my gaze remains focused on it the larger it swells, until it consumes the sky and I begin to slip beneath its tumultuous waters. Unfortunately, because I am human, it often takes me far longer than it should to remember who I am and, more importantly, *whose* I am.

During this particular season it was a year before I suddenly became aware that I was drowning, but the moment I realized my error I shifted my focus off the storm and onto the One who gives hope. It was then that I understood I wasn't being punished for some evil act I had committed, because I am deeply and profoundly loved by my God. As my vision cleared I realized I was on a journey, and that difficulties have a way of shaping and growing us. If we are willing to allow them to run their course we will be better for it in time rather than bitter because of it. The best lessons are often learned during the most difficult seasons. However, there was one particular area of my life I would continue to struggle with in the years that followed.

I knew that if the pain continued to be this intense there was no way I could carry another child. My bladder was in terrible shape as it was, and having a baby pressing on it while being left without any medication to ease the pain seemed too dreadful. I love children; in fact, I believe they are life's greatest gift. For me, there is nothing in this world that compares to the joys of motherhood. Caring for and investing in the lives of my children has given me purpose and profound happiness, and I have never been in a hurry for this phase of life to come to an end. Though my head understood the situation, and I genuinely trusted God with the outcome, the fact that I could not pursue pregnancy seemed to be the biggest blow as I wrestled against my own will and desires.

As each month passed I seemed to sink deeper into a silent depression as further disappointment pushed me below the murky waters. I knew I was struggling to care for the children I had, and that adding to their number would only make things worse. I had experienced difficult pregnancies as it was, and I was afraid of trying to get through another one with these added problems. But I also had a dream of expanding our family and, since motherhood gave me the deepest sense of purpose, the idea of not having more children caused a deep ache that visited me on a recurring basis.

I struggled with the death of my dream for the first five years. We all understand this and have experienced it at some point in our lives. Opening our hands and letting go of something we desperately want can be one of life's most painful experiences. What might have been haunts us in the midst of our unwelcome reality. During these seasons it's important to take a moment to grieve, mourn, and do some quiet soul-searching. But then we must choose to let go. We must accept the new path that presents itself, make the most of our current situation, and press on. Getting trapped in what could have been corrodes the good that still exists, making life bitterly unpleasant for all involved. I am thankful that I was eventually able to get to a place where I was genuinely grateful for what I had as I opened my hands and let go of what could have been. I chose to trust God with my hopes and dreams as I came to understand that if having more children was not His will for my life I had to make my peace with that. I chose to put my trust in Him because I knew He loved me. Once again, the result was profound joy.

As soon as we were unpacked and settled back in San Diego I found a new female urologist, much to my delight. Marianne Rochester is an amazing doctor: warm, kind, sweet, and adventurous. She takes the time to sit and talk with me every time I am there. She shares details and pictures of her travels with me, and never fails to make me laugh. She is a beautiful soul who cares about her patients, and being able to spend a few minutes catching up during each visit is the highlight of my appointments. In fact, I have informed her that she is never allowed to leave her profession unless she wants to find me living in her garage! Choosing her as my doctor brought long-awaited relief from the agonizing pain.

Dr. Rochester began by discussing dimethyl sulfoxide (DMSO) treatments with me, but I was quick to shut her down after my experience with the heparin treatment. This meant delving deeper into the guinea pig era, during which I would try just about every oral option possible. We began with Elavil (amitriptyline).

Chapter 3

THE CLIMB

"Pain is temporary. It may last a minute, or an hour,
or a day, or a year, but eventually it will subside
and something else will take its place.
If I quit, however, it lasts forever."

American cyclist Lance Armstrong

Elavil is an antidepressant, but it is also used to treat chronic nerve pain, as the experts believe it can block nerve signals between the brain and bladder. Though I thought I felt a slight improvement with the Elavil I was still having flare-ups pretty regularly, and on returning to my doctor for another visit we decided to add Atarax (hydroxyzine) to my regimen.

Atarax is an antihistamine and is often used to treat anxiety, but it can also block or hinder the activity of histamine receptors. Along with Elavil and Atarax, we tried using Ultram (tramadol) in place of Vicodin. Ultram is a synthetic opioid, and some people find that they respond to it better than to Vicodin. Of all the medications I have ever used Ultram was by far my least favorite! It caused what I would describe as hallucinations, but since I only took the medicine at night it was really just disrupting my sleep by causing me to have crazy, abnormal dreams that I frequently mistook for reality. I would jump out of bed, freaked out by something I thought I had seen, for example a giant spider the size of the bed. It would take my brain a few moments to catch up before I realized I was dreaming.

I tossed the medicine out after a few nights of that nonsense! In fact, at this point I stopped taking all my medication. I took a break for a while and then decided that, since I still had a bottle of Elmiron, I would give it another go. I also decided to give acupuncture a try. I had it twice a week for a couple of months, which was a huge financial commitment for us at the time, but we had heard that it might help to relieve IC symptoms. It offered no relief whatsoever to my daily pain level, and on the last two occasions I went in it sent me into a major flare-up almost immediately, so I abandoned that as well.

Two weeks after being back on the Elmiron I paid another visit to my doctor and informed her that I was back on it, but that my insurance did not cover the medication, which was expensive. We decided to restart the Atarax, but I began having heart palpitations and stopped using it immediately. In the end, hydrocodone and Pyridium seemed to offer the best relief, though it was always temporary.

IC sufferers can have regular flare-ups, which cause increased pain that is often difficult to manage, even with pain medication. A flare-up can last a few hours or longer, and some left me riddled with pain for more than a week. These were the most difficult to manage, and if the flare-up was particularly bad I found little to no relief in the pain medication. I slept very little at night and would often lie on the floor with a heating pad, which disrupted my husband less (though he never once complained), and honestly felt more comfortable.

My mobility during this time became limited and I often had to clear my schedule so that I could remain at home. After a few days of little sleep and prolonged pain I would lose my appetite, and my emotions often got the best of me as exhaustion took hold. If my bladder was highly irritated I found that I had to resist the urge to bash my head against the wall as I was unable to relieve the chronic irritation. During these times I felt helpless, like I was a burden to my family as I became dependent on them to allow me time to rest. I despised the fact that I was unable to care for them the way my heart longed to. I hated the thought of the drugs running through my system and the fear that, in the end, I would pay a high price for my dependence on them.

Let me just take a moment here to say that even on my worst days I got out of bed and made sure my children had what they needed for the day. It didn't matter how great the pain was or how little I ate or slept, my children's basic needs were always met. It often irritated my body further to get up and move around. There were times when I couldn't even stand up straight and was hunched over as I pushed the shopping cart around Von's, cooked dinner, folded laundry, homeschooled my children, or cleaned up, but I fought through the pain in order to do what needed to be done (albeit not always graciously).

If I needed to be quiet and focus on pushing the tears back, I did. I fought against my body as I sat through countless football and volleyball practices and games, stepping in when needed to serve as team mom, youth leader, hostess, chauffeur, or cheer coach. I made sure we made time to play at the park, do arts and crafts, snuggle, and talk. At the end of the day, it really didn't matter what it cost me. My family always comes first, and as long as I have breath in my lungs I will do what I can to care for those I cherish most in this world. There were many times when my irritability or unusual quietness bore testimony to the pain I was in, but kids deserve to be kids; to play freely without carrying the weight of the world on their shoulders.

I know this may not be a reality for some, as many carry a far greater burden than they should have to. The truth is that life is not fair, but it's what we do in the midst of adversity that matters the most. We must strive to overcome hardship rather than allowing it to permanently derail us, clinging to hope despite our circumstances.

I hate constraints, as I'm certain most of us do, but if you're suffering from chronic pain I want to encourage you to bear your burden as quietly as you can. This doesn't mean that you should lie or pretend everything is fine all the time. It does mean that you should reach deep down inside and find the strength to get up and take care of what you can today without worrying about tomorrow. Choose to put on a brave face when your children are around, and, if you have the ability to meet some of their daily needs, do so as much as possible. If you are married, choose to greet your spouse with a smile each morning and evening. Despite your hardship, make your home a place of refuge for your family; a place of safety that is overflowing with love.

We are far stronger then we think we are, and our ability to endure trials and suffering teaches us, molds us, grows us, and changes us. As humans, we tend to want to flee difficult situations, and we often resent change rather than embracing it. We set up our tents, making sure to nail in the spikes securely, with the subconscious notion that we are safe and cannot be moved. Our comfort zones become our gods as we dig in and refuse to allow change to run its course in making us better humans, spouses, parents, and friends. Trials develop our character, and if we can learn to embrace instead of resisting them we might just be surprised at their ability to make us better, wiser, stronger, more refined people.

I wanted to take the time to discuss our mindset during this chapter because switching gears mentally is a climb in and of itself. But it's a battle to which we ought to dedicate great energy as our thinking can cloud our judgment, deceiving us and stealing our lives away. It has been said that: "We can't always control our circumstances, but we can choose how to respond." There is profound truth in this. What, then, should our attitude be when our world seems to have been turned upside down? How do we find joy amid overwhelming pain or loss? How do we relieve the pain of a broken heart or a shattered dream?

We begin by taking one day at a time; by focusing on today; by focusing on the here and now. The first thing we ought to do is stop fighting change when it is beyond our ability to control it. You have two options when dealing with change: you can either fight against it, which will make you miserable as you wrestle against your will and reality; or you can choose to accept it and allow it to run its course, changing you from the inside out. Change is a natural part of life, and it provides the opportunity to broaden our horizons, develop our character, and soften our hearts.

Part of the reason we despise change is that we are afraid the journey will lead us somewhere we don't want to go. A fear of the unknown keeps us on the shore when we were created to sail on its waters. We often allow ourselves to succumb to fear (fear of the unknown, of change, or of a difficult or uncomfortable situation), which renders us ineffectual. Putting fear in its rightful place is no easy task, but it is a necessary step if we ever hope to get out from under its tyrannical hand.

Fear tells us we can't handle the situation; that we will never get through this heartbreak unscathed; that a certain fear will come to pass, and we won't be able to bear it. Motives and desires are often birthed out of fear, but fear deceives us and often leads to a pessimistic attitude, whereby we focus on the negatives of life rather than the joys of living it. Reigning fear dims our vision, and as a result we lose our ability to clearly see what is right in front of us. This causes us to make poor decisions based on our limited visibility and convoluted mindsets, as we are no longer able to properly assess our situations in the full light of reality.

We all have fears we must contend with, and if we are not careful we may unconsciously go through life projecting those feelings onto others. If we are afraid of losing a child we may hold them too close, never affording them the freedom to spread their wings. If we fear heartbreak we may not allow anyone to come too close, let alone have our heart. The fear of poverty may drive someone to become a workaholic, while the need to be in charge in case things do not unfold the way we desire may cause another to become a control freak. Fear of failure may keep you from taking risks, convincing you that you can't step out and try something new, and closing the door on your dreams. Or you may fear that life will always be lived with the severe pain related to IC, and that you are beyond hope; forever weighed down by this incredible burden and unable to gather enough strength to fight your way back.

There are things we can control and things we can't, and we need to know the difference. The things we are unable to control can be given to God each morning, because He loves us and can be trusted with our hopes and dreams. Let go of the things you were never meant to take ownership of, then choose to face your fears head on and with great courage.

Nelson Mandela once said: "I learned that courage was not the absence of fear, but the triumph over it. The brave man is not he who does not feel afraid, but he who conquers that fear."

We all have fears. Some are rational and others are irrational, but in order to overcome them we must choose to proceed with courage. It is the positivity of our thoughts, the openness of our hearts, and the willingness of our spirits that will determine the way we behave and enable us to face all that life can throw at us rather than leaving us chained to a post or even to our past. Of course, we must understand that not all fear is irrational. Rational fear has its place, after all. We will not get through this life without ever facing momentary situations when we or someone we love is in clear and immediate danger. But more often than not we find that we are struggling with irrational fear, which is based on emotion, misperception, and exaggeration.

Have you ever stopped to think how different your life would be if fear were removed from the equation? If you had no fear to contend with, what would you be doing right now? What risks would you take? What adventure would you take off on? How deeply would you love? I am terrified of heights and sharks, but let's focus on one thing at a time! I have begun facing my fear of heights as the opportunities present themselves; choosing to climb, fly, jump, or take a zip line through the jungle whenever I'm given the chance. Fear creeps up inside me in each of these situations, causing my heart to race, my body to stiffen, my toes to go numb, and my mind to run through every horrifying scenario possible. I know that, in this moment, I have to choose to put one foot in front of the other, moving right toward the thing I am most afraid of. Otherwise, rather than moving forward I will most certainly fall back, wasting a perfectly good opportunity to exert my courage in light of the fear that fills me.

You see, fear only has the power we give it, so let's offer it little room in our minds so that it can't rob us of the lives we were meant to live. It's not necessarily about being fearless; it's about choosing to be brave and courageous when staring fear in the face, rather than choosing to rest in its embrace.

Mark Twain said: "Courage is resistance to fear, mastery of fear – not absence of fear." Let's choose to be courageous men and women who navigate through life refusing to be walled in by fear and the deception that travels alongside it. If left unchecked it will certainly direct our course.

We can also control our attitudes and approach. We can choose to have hope despite the grim outlook, and to fight instead of shutting down and checking out. We can choose to be selfish and self-centered, making it all about us and how we feel, or we can choose to be selfless, putting the interests of others before ourselves. We make these choices every single day! We must repeatedly choose to respond to the difficulties in our lives with grace, strength, and great courage. Show up, be present, fight when you feel like giving in, push on even though you're tired, and stand firm instead of compromising. You are responsible for your actions, your thoughts, and your choices. Take responsibility for them and, when necessary, make amends.

Choosing to think positively will affect your daily life, so be intentional about where you choose to set your mind each moment of every day. Fill your world with beauty, encouraging quotes (I write them on Post-it notes and stick them around the house, or on my bathroom mirror, or in my journal), good books, and Bible verses. Spend time with friends who encourage you, and don't tear you or anyone else down. Watch TV shows or movies that lift your spirit, or listen to beautiful music. Sit outside and let the warmth of the sun remind you that you were created for a reason, and that your life has a purpose. Give time to the things that make you smile and warm your heart, and be thankful despite your situation, counting your blessings every day. I am learning to let go of the things I can't control, and am focusing instead on loving deeply, fiercely, and without condition.

We all have dreams and ideas about how life should be, or at least how life was supposed to be, and most of us have held certain ideals for as long as we can remember. Oftentimes, life doesn't turn out as we had hoped, dreamed, or planned. It throws us curveballs, crushing our dreams while leaving us dazed and confused. If we are not careful in guarding our hearts we can grow bitter and resentful, especially when we look at those around us who seem to have been dealt a far better hand in life than we have.

Don't compare yourself to anyone else! You are your own person: beautiful, smart, strong, and courageous. Comparing yourself to others and measuring your success in view of theirs will leave you miserable and unfulfilled. Joy comes when we are grateful for what we have, and when we learn to make the most of every opportunity. One of the best ways to do this is by learning to focus on others rather on ourselves. Selfishness is ugly. It doesn't look good on anyone, no matter how expensive the outfit. Choose to give your time, talents, money, energy, and love to those who need it, and when you take stock of all you have you will find that you are rich and deeply blessed in the things that matter most. New dreams will grow in the soil where old ones have died, and the flowers that eventually spring up in that soil will fill your life with more beauty and color than you ever could have imagined.

Perhaps one of the most vital necessities in life is the ability to forgive; refusing to hold grudges because we know that unforgiveness grows roots of bitterness, resentment, insecurity, negativity, and hatred. It spreads like cancer within us, robbing us of all that is good. When we choose to forgive others we are set free from the chains that once held us captive. It is in the act of forgiving one another that we let go of the past and move forward, allowing for growth and healing to begin; laying a firm foundation in order to build something new and beautiful in its place. Forgiveness provides the opportunity for transformation, healing, restoration, and, where possible, reconciliation.

What legacy will you leave when your time has come to depart this earth? Forgiving those who have wronged, abused, rejected, or abandoned you is a choice. Extending forgiveness is a gift rooted in a love that refuses to keep a record of every wrong because it understands that, even on our best day, we too fall short. We are all human, flawed, and selfish. Forgiveness restores hope within, allows healing to begin, and releases us from a victim mentality. It leaves the past... in the past. It opens the gates so that love can flow freely, changing the legacy we leave our families and the generations that follow. Your freedom and mine is found in our ability to forgive one another.

Finally, understand that in order to get your health back you will have to be patient as you fight against this condition. You will struggle in your body, in your flesh, and in your mind. Your body is sick, and it is screaming at you, loudly. Your flesh wants what it wants and is rarely, if ever, satisfied by anything life has to offer. Your mind will have moments and days when it is worn down, when your judgment is clouded. You may feel as though you lack the willpower to push on.

In these moments, and in the days ahead, you must resolve to walk in wisdom and self-control, and to fight against it all. You must learn to listen to your body. It is speaking to you, so pay attention. Our flesh needs to be checked and we must take authority over it. There have been moments when I have been in the middle of a flare-up, feeling completely worn down, yet my flesh wants Starbucks. I justify giving it what it wants because I'm already in pain, and I want it. I don't care what's best for me in that moment, because I want it. I know that it will make me temporarily happy, and I want it. And lastly, I want it. I know it's not wise and that I'll pay for it later, but I don't care because I want what I want, when I want it.

We need to practice telling our flesh no, and refusing to give in to its incessant cravings and demands. Our emotions cannot be trusted, and we must be able to identify the traitor within that desperately tries to deceive us and lead us astray. Wisdom whispers truth to us throughout the day, but we often pretend we can't hear her. Wisdom tells me that my fancy Starbucks drink is unwise, unhealthy, acidic, and full of chemicals that will not only irritate my bladder but will have long-term consequences. I have begun to practice the art of listening, so that when wisdom whispers I refuse to ignore her, unwilling to bend to every craving of my flesh.

I refuse to close my eyes and pretend that what I eat and drink will have no real effect on my quality of life. I choose to read, research, study, and – most importantly – apply what I have learned. I am intentional about how I live my life, and I am a fighter! There are days when I am weak and compromise in areas I shouldn't, but those days are becoming far less frequent. And if I fail I can hope in my tomorrow, for tomorrow is a new day, and it offers a fresh start. The more I apply what I have learned with regard to my health, the healthier my body feels. It doesn't come overnight, but neither did the IC. It is one step after another of refusing to quit, compromise, or play the fool.

Lastly, accept that IC brings some limitations and make your peace with it. Find joy despite your situation, and strive to live life to the fullest. A few years into my life with IC I made a new friend who would end up impacting my life and pushing me into a new season. Paige and I met at a Bible study group she was leading at the time. She is a beautiful person inside and out; my dearest friend, and a constant encouragement. She was training for a marathon when we met and was committed to reaching her goal. Her dedication had a profound effect on me and I wanted to join her, but I knew that I couldn't physically handle the jogging. I could hardly walk a block, let alone jog it, and I felt discouraged. But because of Paige's commitment to training I also felt inspired.

One day, something on the inside shifted yet again. I knew what I wanted, and I was willing to endure the uphill battle in order to reach my goal. I decided it was time to get in shape! I knew I was done sitting at home in pain. I wanted to begin working out, but my body felt weak, slow, and tired. As I thought about the pain that constantly erupted when I walked, I figured it had to be due, at least in part, to the fact that I was using my core muscles to move around, and when those core muscles tightened they placed pressure on my bladder, causing it to become more irritated. My logic was that if I slowly strengthened those muscles they would eventually become stronger and able to endure more strenuous activity. I set a goal. I wanted to be able to jog a mile, and I gave myself a year to do it.

I began with walking a single block.

Chapter 4

A NEW SEASON

"If we had no winter, the spring would not be so pleasant; if we did not sometimes taste of adversity, prosperity would not be so welcome."

English poet Anne Bradstreet

Over the next few months, walking a single block turned into a couple miles. I even picked up a Pilates video and began using it regularly at home. The kids often walked with me, and it became a beautiful time to share together. We would talk and laugh, then stop by the local coffee shop and share a smoothie.

The pain that accompanied each new phase of exercise was often brutal, but I would put my focus elsewhere so that it didn't consume me. There were many times as I struggled against my body that I would audibly yell as I took authority over it. I knew that IC wouldn't kill me, so I pushed myself to do what became an almost everyday activity. A few months passed and I began to throw quick sprints into my walks. At first I could hardly run twenty-five yards, but I kept on pushing, and would often scream at my body: "Shut up and do what I say!"

I felt alive and invigorated! My body was getting stronger, and so was my mind. Hope was in full bloom, and I was excited to see the progress I had made. But although I was doing more than I ever had since becoming sick, the constant pain was still there. During this season my urologist finally wore me down and I decided to give the DMSO treatments a try. After all, I had tried just about everything else, and she was hopeful that I would see good results.

I only had a vague recollection of what the first treatment would entail, but it was enough to make me nervous. A catheter was inserted and my bladder was drained. Next I was given lidocaine, a local anesthetic, and then the DMSO cocktail. My urologist instructed me to try to hold it for five minutes, which I assumed would be a piece of cake, and then I could go to the restroom. The five minutes seemed more than doable when she was explaining the process, but the second the DMSO was inserted into my bladder it felt like someone had lit a match inside me. My husband had to pin me down until the five minutes were up. It was awful!

When Tom finally let me up I made a mad dash for the bathroom. The moment I was done urinating the stinging spiked, and I struggled to fight back the tears. I sobbed most of the way home, but fortunately the pain had dwindled by the time we got there. Shortly after arriving home I felt the urge to urinate, and I became increasingly afraid and stressed out. I held off as long as I could, then sat on the toilet crying and trembling. My sweet husband stood in front of me, holding me and assuring me it was going to be OK. After a couple of minutes I finally relaxed enough to go, but the second the urine hit my urethra it felt like a knife had been inserted into me. My sobbing grew louder, my trembling stronger. I crawled into bed and waited desperately for the pain to die down again. I spent the remainder of the day in bed.

I was to come back once a week for the next six to eight weeks for treatments, and the goal was to eventually hold the DMSO for twenty minutes each time. After the treatments we would evaluate my progress to see if there had been any improvement.

The following week I cried on the way to the doctor's office as the mere thought of the pain scared me. I detested the treatments and hated my body every single week. After a couple of sessions my doctor let me know that I could take hydrocodone and Pyridium before coming in. She also used a little extra lidocaine during the treatment, as well as the smallest catheter she had. This helped tremendously with the treatments, and I was beyond grateful.

However, every time I left her office and reached the car the pain surged, and I would climb in, crying and tense. The thirty-minute drive home was brutal, and all I could think about was how much I just wanted to get into bed and lie down with my heating pad. My kids were amazing on treatment days, and I was greeted with my heating pad warmed up, a grilled cheese sandwich with a side of baby carrots, and an episode of *Friends*. Then they let me sleep until the pain had quieted down.

After six treatments I saw a slight improvement, albeit short-lived. At the time of my ninth treatment the doctor suggested we extend to twelve sessions and then re-evaluate. If, after twelve, I hadn't seen a significant improvement we would abandon the DMSO treatments altogether. She was as surprised as I was that I wasn't seeing more of an improvement, and I didn't know what it meant for me in the long run. I felt extremely disappointed.

However, after treatment ten I began to feel a slight relief from the daily pain, so we reduced the treatments to every other week. We were eventually able to spread them out even further, and I began to only need them every four weeks or so.

Around the time of treatments fifteen and sixteen the DMSO seemed to lose its effect on my body, so my doctor decided to try a heparin treatment. The first left me riddled with pain. I got home, went to my room where I could be alone, and sobbed. The pain overwhelmed me as I crouched in the corner of the room crying, hugging my knees, and rocking back and forth in a desperate attempt to soothe my trembling body. At the following appointment I agreed to give it one more try, then I swore off heparin treatments forever and went back to DMSO. I eventually got to a place where I was averaging six to eight weeks between treatments, and I loved that I was regaining part of my life.

At times I could go beyond the eight weeks between treatments, and was functioning at seventy percent of "normal" health. The pain was still there, and I had to use hydrocodone at night to help me sleep through it, but I began to feel like I was getting stronger.

One day while I was out exercising I decided to give in to temptation and run the stairs at the park. I pushed myself but felt invigorated, and I smiled as each step passed by beneath me. On the walk home I felt elated. The sky appeared bluer and the trees looked greener. Unfortunately, my bladder was in a tremendous amount of pain by nightfall, and I was shocked at the sight of blood when I went to the restroom. I had heard that IC patients can suffer from hematuria, but this was my first experience of a bladder bleed.

It certainly wasn't my last. Whenever I experienced bleeding the pain was far worse than at any other time, and I felt like a wounded animal, curled up and whimpering. Because the DMSO appeared to be working I was pushing my body further and harder, as I couldn't necessarily feel the pain in that moment. This resulted in my bladder becoming irritated to such an extent that it bled. Wisdom told me to back down with regard to my exercise routine, but my determination to reach my goals foolishly pushed me on.

A little more than two years had passed since beginning the DMSO treatments. I worried about the medicine running through my system, and the continual use of the catheter made me fear that my bladder would suffer permanent scarring. On the bright side, I had lost ten pounds. By the time I was almost thirty-six I felt stronger and could handle a light sixty-minute workout. I began to notice that my body was struggling somewhat, but I wasn't exactly sure what was going on.

At lunch one afternoon a group of friends shared their opinion that it was most likely a hormone imbalance. A couple of friends recommended a doctor who took a more natural approach to health than is common in Western medicine. I made the appointment, but had no idea that walking into this next doctor's office would mark the beginning of a completely new season in my life.

Donald Adema, D.O., treated me for a couple of issues, namely hormone imbalance and adrenal fatigue. He also tested me for the MTHFR gene mutation. MTHFR is a gene that provides specific instructions for an enzyme called methylenetetrahydrofolate. This enzyme plays a role in processing amino acids and chemical reactions in the body, including an important metabolic process called methylation. A defect in this gene can impact the way your body metabolizes folate and folic acid. My results showed that I possessed the MTHFR gene mutation A1298C, and Dr. Adema began treating me with methylated B12 and folate shots that very afternoon. The first shot sent me into a major flare-up within an hour, so we reduced the dosage by half the following week. I began going in weekly for the shot, and by the third week my bladder seemed to be quieting down. I went in for a DMSO treatment around this time, but little did I know that it would be my last one!

Dr. Adema believed the B12 and folate could possibly help with the chronic inflammation, but we were both surprised at how well I responded. I eventually increased the dosage and then began giving myself the shot at home to save money. The results were staggering, and after a few months I was functioning at eighty-five percent. I was getting my life back!

I am beyond grateful for everything Dr. Adema did for me, and for the constant encouragement and support he offered me and my family. At that point in my journey with IC I was doing extremely well, but I was still dealing with mild daily irritation and sporadic flare-ups. I knew I was close to understanding this illness, and I desperately wanted to close the gap that remained between where I was and finally sending my IC into remission. The peak of the mountain was so close that I could almost touch it, so I pressed on and continued reading and studying in desperate search of answers.

I forged on with my own research and documentation so I could get clarity as to what had caused my IC and what was continuing to contribute to my symptoms. However, I could never have fully understood what was going on without the help, direction, and input of Patricia Deckert, D.O. She opened up a world of genetics to me and impressed upon me the significant role it would play in the future of medicine.

Though I started to see significant improvement in my IC symptoms when I started the B12 and folate shots, Dr. Deckert and I understand that this was not the best place to start when addressing inflammatory illnesses or autoimmune conditions. The best place to start when dealing with any health issue is to get to the root cause. Modern medicine focuses on treating symptoms, which is not the same as getting the root of the issue. Something was causing the chronic inflammation, so I needed to figure out what it was and address it head on.

PART 2

Chapter 5

TIME TO DETOX

"We are all faced with a series of great opportunities –
brilliantly disguised as insoluble problems."

American educator, author, and activist
John W. Gardner

In this day and age it's hard to safeguard your body from toxins. They're in the air we breathe, the food we eat, and the products we use to clean our homes. As much as we try to limit our exposure to toxins and live healthy lifestyles, it's often unavoidable. But while this may be a challenge, reducing our exposure to toxins is essential if we want to live healthy lives.

Overexposure to toxins can have a negative effect on our bodies. When everything from environmental toxins and pesticides to harmful chemicals and heavy metals get stored in our tissues and cells it can traumatize our bodies. This may affect metabolism, immune system, behavior, and overall health. Toxins disrupt the body's natural balance, which can ultimately lead to illness. While all humans neutralize and excrete toxins to a certain extent, the level to which our bodies are able to eradicate them depends on various factors, including genetics, underlying health issues, liver function, methylation rates, diet, and lifestyle.

Take my garbage disposal as an example. When it works, it makes life a little easier. I can pulverize food scraps, and with the help of running water pushing the contents out into the waste line I don't have to worry about clogging my pipes. But when it's backed up and nothing can get through, life suddenly seems so much harder.

I was recently washing my dishes when this very dilemma struck. My garbage disposal was full and started backing up into the sink. I tried to flip the switch, but nothing happened. Then I tried the reset button. I thought if I could at least stop the flow of electricity the unit wouldn't overload and break. But again, that did nothing. Too much waste had coated the drain trap or pipe, causing a clog. Of course, it could also have been caused by someone (not me, of course) sticking something into the disposal that didn't belong there. At a loss, I called my brilliant husband who looked at the unit with a wrench and a flashlight, and promptly confirmed my worst fear: the garbage disposal would need to be replaced. However, since it was the time of the Olympics I would have to wait – with my sink full of junk – until the following day for him to replace it!

This is similar to the way the human body works. If too many toxins build up inside us and overload our systems our bodies are no longer able to cope. They essentially malfunction, laying the groundwork for dysfunction and illness. If we aren't able to properly dispose of the toxins our systems get clogged. Just like my waste disposal system, we need to remove the clogs, unjam the unit, clear the buildup, reset the system, and run water through it to resolve the issue.

You don't have to look farther than interstitial cystitis to see what happens when our bodies struggle to effectively rid themselves of toxins. The turning point in my journey came when I finally and fully understood the toxic state I had been living in. I decided to undergo a metabolic detox to rid my body of toxic overload, reset my system, and restore my body's natural balance.

My cleanse of choice was the Metabolic Detox UltraClear Plus pH from Metagenics: a twenty-eight-day, science-based program that works to rid the body of harmful toxins and chemicals. In my case, the results were dramatic. I started to notice a difference after just three days. For the first time in ten years I no longer felt pain in my bladder. It was a game-changer for me. I decided on the twenty-eight-day detox over the ten-day option because of the severity of my IC, as well as taking into account the fact that I had been sick for a decade. A ten-day option is available, so speak with your doctor or nutritionist and they will guide you.

The Metagenics program is designed to enhance the body's natural metabolic detoxification via a three-phase process (Phase I, Phase II, and Phase III). It breaks down toxins and makes them more water-soluble, so the body can eventually excrete them. With the cleanse, you receive UltraClear Plus pH: a rice protein powder that is specially designed to enhance the detoxification process. It uses macro- and micronutrients to address liver function, while providing all the full energy you need. Additionally, the pH formula promotes alkalization. The program also comes with AdvaClear: supplements that deliver vitamins and minerals to help support detoxification while offering antioxidant support.

The Metagenics detox fills in the gaps left by juice cleanses and so many other detox methods out there. Instead of simply limiting what your body takes in, Metagenics provides the extra nutritional support you need to feel better. I love this because rather than leaving you feeling hungry or tired, it fills you with the best fuel your body can get. Detoxing should be carried out safely so toxins can be eliminated effectively while restoring nutrient and metabolic balance.

While I first looked into undertaking a metabolic detox in response to my struggle with interstitial cystitis, I learned that many people choose to undertake a cleanse several times a year. This form of regular "spring cleaning" can help get you back on track to a healthier lifestyle.

A quick visit to the Metagenics website will point you in the direction of a doctor or nutritionist near you who can support you through the cleanse. There are also metabolic detoxification questionnaires you can take to assess whether it's right for you. Other nutraceutical companies that offer quality detox kits are Orthomolecular and Xymogen. Sara Gottfried, M.D., Alan Christiansen, N.M.D., and Mark Hyman, M.D., offer a range of online resources to guide you toward the right detox program for you.

Whichever detox option you choose, it's important to pick one that lasts a minimum of seven days. During this time the diet should always be limited. Each one varies, but most eliminate dairy, citrus, sugar, caffeine, alcohol, gluten, and some other grains. The reasoning behind this is that many of these are allergens and can trigger inflammation. It is usually recommended that you consume only low-glycemic fruits and vegetables, including: artichokes, asparagus, bean sprouts, broccoli, cauliflower, celery, cucumber, leeks, microgreens, radishes, squash, Swiss chard, cabbage, zucchini, cherries, prunes, apples, pears, strawberries, and peaches. You should also eat high-quality proteins such as freshly caught fish, organic fowl and grass-fed beef, along with more exotic meats. Nearly all pathways are dependent on adequate levels of healthy protein being present in order to eliminate toxins.

The reasons for detoxing vary but should always stem from a desire to feel better. Symptoms that may improve following a detox include fatigue, low mood, brain fog, digestive issues, allergic symptoms, and inflammatory conditions such as interstitial cystitis. The most important reasons to carry out a detox is to clean up the diet, support liver function, rid the body of toxins, and break addictions and cravings. It is then much easier to introduce a healthy diet and stick to it in order to achieve your long-term healthcare goals. An additional benefit for some may be weight loss. Reducing toxic burden can speed up the metabolism, making a healthy diet work more efficiently and making weight loss goals more achievable.

If you're just starting out on your journey toward a healthier you a detox is a good first step. You'll be amazed at what a natural recharge can do for your body, mind, and soul.

Understanding the role of the liver

A metabolic detox will support liver function, but it may be necessary to offer this important organ additional support once you are done detoxifying. Poor liver function leads to an inability to detoxify, which is what I believe played a key role in me – and probably you – developing IC.

The liver is the largest solid organ in your body, and it carries out more than 500 functions that are critical to your wellbeing. At the top of that list is detoxification. It can filter a liter of blood per minute and produce up to 1.5 quarters of bile every day. Bile helps our bodies break down fat from food so that we can more easily digest it. This crucial organ takes all the harmful toxins that have entered our bloodstream, whether through the environment, chemicals, drugs or heavy metals, and turns them into bile so they can be eliminated. It also helps keep our hormones and blood sugar levels balanced so we can function properly.

The liver is our gatekeeper to better health, but because of its important role it is often under enormous stress. Whether we overburden it with poor-quality food, toxins, chemicals, or conditions such as interstitial cystitis, the liver is one of the hardest-working organs in our body. Give it too much work to do and it may become unable to cope.

Several conditions that affect the immune system are caused by this breakdown. Issues such as allergies, autoimmune disorders, and even certain types of arthritis can be significantly reduced if enough attention is dedicated to keeping the liver healthy. When the liver is unable to do its job properly it cannot keep out all the dangerous toxins or undigested food particles. When these foreign objects are allowed to travel deeper and deeper into your body, the risk they pose increases. This can lead to asthma, eczema, and certain types of cancer if the damage to your cells is great enough.

Additionally, an underperforming liver can lead to a weakened immune system. The body may struggle to respond, and the effects can be widespread. It may start to secrete mast cells and release histamine. This is what ultimately leads to pain and inflammation. While the liver naturally produces antihistamines, its capacity will be diminished if it is under too much stress. Symptoms of interstitial cystitis and other autoimmune conditions will persist for as long as the liver is weak and normal function is impaired.

The good news is that once you start paying more attention to your liver you should start to see an improvement in your symptoms. Through cleansing, detoxifying, and supporting your liver with essential nutrients your liver can regain its strength, restore its ability to detoxify your body, and start to produce antihistamines again. The most encouraging notion here is the liver's ability to regenerate. That's because it possesses a high capacity for regeneration, far exceeding that of any other organ in the body.

This is good news for us because it means that we can support the liver through the regeneration process so that it can repair damaged tissue with new cells. Regeneration only takes a few weeks, but it is imperative that you remove toxins, eat healthily, and reduce alcohol consumption. A competent liver will completely detoxify any mast-cell triggers – neutralizing drugs, toxins, and additives, and combating estrogen build-up, for example – and will start producing natural antihistamines again.

When we talk about removing toxins, this includes not only chemicals present in household cleaning products, skincare, cookware, and water, but also in pain meds. Allow me to explain. I understand the pain, and believe me I support our access to these medications. When IC pain is so intolerable that you want to pull your hair out or bash your head against a wall you need to have the option to self-medicate. During the healing process you'll want to find natural remedies to treat pain and inflammation, but let's be honest; they don't always work immediately when the pain is severe.

Medicine has its place and I am grateful for it. Any time I got sick with a cold or the flu, or accidently ate something I was intolerant to, or had a UTI, it would always increase my IC symptoms. I am grateful that I had access to pain meds on those occasions when my pain was intolerable. It is cruel to leave someone in that much pain and refuse them relief. However, what I came to understand about pain medication is that it increases oxidative stress, which in turn causes inflammation! It becomes a vicious cycle and we have to get off the hamster wheel if we ever hope to regain our health. Pain medications also negatively affect the liver and digestive tract. When trying to bring the body into balance you need to be vigilant about protecting it from toxins, and pain meds are toxic to the body. Proceed with caution and seek natural remedies whenever possible in order to thwart inflammation. Oil of oregano (a natural antibiotic), probiotics (which support healthy gut flora), herbal teas, and certain supplements can offer relief without the side-effects.

If you feel you need additional liver support after you have completed the metabolic detox, speak with your doctor about the best means of going about this. There are a number of options available, from liver support supplements and natural liver detoxes and cleanses, to a liver and gallbladder flush. These treatments go by different names, but the goal is the same. If you do decide to embark upon a liver detox make sure you do your due diligence because some may exacerbate IC symptoms and you certainly don't want to do that. Whichever option you choose it should be gentle on your system as it supports your body's natural ability to detoxify itself.

Chapter 6

IT'S A GUT THING

"Every strike brings me closer to the next home run."

American baseball player Babe Ruth

It's interesting that IC appears among the American Autoimmune Related Diseases Association's list of eighty-eight known autoimmune-related conditions. This is intriguing because at this stage I had not yet come across anyone who had looked at my IC through the lens of autoimmunity, and therefore no attempt had been made to evaluate and determine where I was on the autoimmune spectrum, let alone to address the root cause of my chronic inflammation. This lack of knowledge made closing the gap impossible until now.

Sending IC into remission may not be possible for some if the obstacles that are interfering with the immune system's ability to function are not addressed and removed. This new revelation got me thinking that perhaps the best way to get to the bottom of things was to make an appointment with an integrative or functional medicine practitioner.

Integrative or functional medicine looks at the body as a whole, taking a system-oriented approach. This is a completely different method from the one taken by those practicing conventional or traditional medicine. In most cases the latter take a disease-centered focus and treat only the symptoms. If we hope to regain our health we cannot simply isolate the bladder, focusing solely on this organ. We must view the body in its entirety.

Having the right doctor makes all the difference, believe me! Find a reputable integrative, functional, naturopathic, or holistic doctor who can come alongside and walk this road with you until you are well on the road to recovery. Dr. Deckert has brought knowledge and insight to areas I could never have uncovered on my own, and I am beyond thankful that our paths crossed because she has been a tremendous blessing in my life, the quality of which has drastically improved since.

Few of us truly understand just how important and influential our immune systems are. Protecting us day and night, they can detect a whole load of pathogens, including bacteria, viruses, and parasites. The immune system is clever enough to easily distinguish between these unwanted invaders and the body's own healthy tissue. It really is our first line of defense against infection and disease.

In light of this, we need to keep our immune systems healthy and strong so they continue to create this vital barrier between our bodies and the toxins we're exposed to in everyday life. Keeping our immune systems healthy helps to ensure that harmful pathogens are detected and destroyed before we even begin to experience any ill effects.

In addition, a strong and healthy immune system will help to control inflammation levels in the body. The goal is to maintain a zero-inflammation level, but if the immune system is weak our inflammation levels can rise. The type of chronic inflammation I have experienced with IC is a clear indication that the immune system is overworked and under extreme pressure. Chronic inflammation can trigger an autoimmune condition, and if the inflammation is not reduced and the root cause eliminated any symptoms will grow worse and your health will continue to decline. This explains why those with IC may also have IBS, fibromyalgia, vulvodynia, ulcerative colitis, chronic fatigue, prostatitis, and other such conditions. In extreme cases the immune system becomes overburdened and ends up "going rogue," starting to attack healthy tissue. This is a recipe for disaster and can have long-lasting and extremely debilitating effects.

Understanding that my IC could develop into a full-blown autoimmune disease if I didn't get a handle on it was a real eye-opener for me. Many people with chronic inflammation – including those with IC – believe that if we can keep our inflammation under control, for example the symptoms of our asthma, bladder inflammation, acne, arthritis, or skin rashes, we can simply continue on down the road to which we have grown accustomed. The truth is, if our immune systems are on heightened alert and chronic inflammation is our reality, the only option we have is to get to the root of it all or risk further illness. This begins with identifying the threat that is keeping the immune system on permanent alert.

A healthy gut means a healthy immune system

Did you know that the gut accounts for eighty percent of the body's immune system? As such, a healthy gut equals a strong immune system. The truth is that our bodies are made up of many different systems that must work together effectively if we want to stay healthy. If one of these systems is out of sync this can have a domino effect on other areas of the body. Another system is affected, then another and another. Before long our bodies are in meltdown and we have a whole range of new chronic health conditions to battle.

Your gut and immune system work particularly closely, so if your gut is unhealthy your immune system will undoubtedly begin to struggle. As the gut is often the first point of entry for toxins, it's vital it is in a good condition so that it acts as a barrier to prevent disease. Should its complex network of cells, proteins, tissues, and organs become compromised it's likely that your whole immune system will become rundown, allowing harmful bacteria to thrive and attack the body.

Most of our digestion takes place in the small intestine, so making sure this part of the gastrointestinal (GI) tract is healthy and functioning properly is vital. Inside the small intestine is a brush border, which is made up of small, finger-like projections called "villi," which are covered in "microvilli" that look like tiny hairs. Used in combination, this increases the surface area of the gut to roughly the size of a tennis court, allowing for better absorption of nutrients. This brush border sweeps nutrients from our food into the gut and directs them toward the epithelial wall (the single-cell layer that forms the lining of both the small and large intestine), which only allows the smallest molecules to pass through the intestinal wall and into the bloodstream. At the same time, it works hard to keep harmful substances out.

Once in the bloodstream, nutrients are carried throughout the body, providing it with the nourishment it needs to function correctly. The epithelial wall is made up of enterocytes and held together by tight junctions. The term "tight junctions" is important here. It is only one cell thick, but the gut lining accounts for the body's largest cluster of protective cell layers. Maintaining the integrity of this barrier correlates directly with the condition of the GI tract, immune system, endocrine system, and nervous system. Suffice to say, it's worth keeping an eye on!

When the tight junctions begin to come apart (known as "leaky gut" or intestinal permeability), toxins, undigested food, and unfriendly microbes are able to breach the barrier and enter the bloodstream, to our detriment. Leaky gut diminishes the small intestine's ability to absorb nutrients because damage to the villi and microvilli reduces the surface area of the small intestine. This means that even if we're eating a healthy diet we may not be reaping the full benefits nutritionally. Once leaky gut is in play we begin to have a host of other issues to contend with because, as the name suggests, it also causes the walls of the intestines to leak. As toxic invaders that have no business entering our bloodstream find their way in, the immune system fires up and begins producing inflammatory chemicals in response, creating extra antibodies to fight against these invaders.

The immune system comprises a collection of structures and processes, including lymph nodes, the spleen, bone marrow, lymphocytes, thymus, and leukocytes. Designed to protect us against disease and dangerous foreign bodies, the immune system takes on two roles: "innate" and "adaptive." The innate immune system responds immediately to a threat and possesses no memory, so it maintains no history of immunity. Once invaders enter the bloodstream the innate immune system responds with acute inflammation as it starts releasing inflammatory chemicals (antibodies) in an all-out effort to protect us.

This is what happens when we get the flu, for example. Inflammation, which can be painful, kicks up in our nasal passages and our bodies feel achy, swollen, tired, and hot as our immune systems work hard to defeat the bugs. Once the enemy is defeated the inflammation dies back down, and all is well again. The immune system then returns to its normal resting state.

By contrast, our adaptive immune systems have a slower response. The adaptive immune system develops over time and retains information beyond the invader's lifespan, creating a form of resistance that may last a lifetime. This is why immunizations work to protect us from infectious diseases such as polio or measles, as they provide us with long-term immunity.

Signs you may have leaky gut

When leaky gut becomes an issue, the adaptive immune system stays on high alert and continues to fire off inflammatory chemicals at a whole host of invaders as they enter the bloodstream. Examples of potential invaders (though these do not affect everyone in the same way) may include gluten, dairy, eggs, soy, peanuts, and refined sugar. As you continue to eat these inflammation-causing foods day in and day out, the immune system becomes overloaded in its constant all-out attempt to defeat them, and acute inflammation evolves into chronic inflammation.

How do you know if you have leaky gut? If you have an autoimmune disease or condition it's fairly safe to say that you have leaky gut. Many functional medicine doctors now believe that leaky gut is behind a number of diseases that are specific to first-world nations.

The following symptoms most likely point to leaky gut:

- Chronic inflammation (for example IC, arthritis or Crohn's disease)
- Osteoporosis (fragile bones)
- Mood issues (such as depression, anxiety, panic attacks, and stress)
- Brain fog (for example confusion, difficulty concentrating, and memory loss)
- Digestive system issues (such as acid reflux, IBS, bloating, constipation, and diarrhea)
- Hormone imbalance (too much or too little of our natural hormones, for example progesterone, testosterone, and cortisol)
- Chronic fatigue
- Frequent colds or infections
- Food intolerance or sensitivity
- Muscle and joint pain
- Candida (thrush, recurring yeast infections, jock itch)
- Small intestinal bacterial overgrowth (SIBO)
- Skin issues (acne, eczema, psoriasis, rashes, and athlete's foot)
- Low metabolism
- Nutrient deficiency

With the American diet being as it is, added to our constant exposure to toxins, it is believed that a significant proportion of people in the U.S. suffer from leaky gut. Some experts believe that as many as eighty percent of us may have it! With millions of Americans suffering from gastrointestinal issues, it is important to identify the underlying conditions that could be responsible for an attack on our digestive systems.

Furthermore, when leaky gut is in play it more often than not brings unwelcome friends along with it including SIBO, candida overgrowth, and irritable bowel syndrome (IBS). Many people with IC also struggle with candida overgrowth, which causes chronic yeast infections, and many also suffer with IBS. We will take a minute to explore these issues, but the good news is that whether you are addressing one or all of them the course of action is basically the same.

SIBO

If you often suffer from bloating or gas, or you regularly have diarrhea, constipation, inflammatory bowel disease (IBD), vitamin and mineral deficiencies, IBS, autoimmune disease, hypothyroidism, acid reflux, or joint pain, you could be suffering from an infection in your gut. An imbalance in the bacteria present can result in what is known as small intestinal bacterial overgrowth (SIBO). According to Dr. Amy Myers, forty percent of people have been misdiagnosed with IBS when they actually have SIBO.

In a healthy person, the small intestine will usually contain low levels of bacteria compared with other parts of the body. This is where the nutrients are pulled from your food and absorbed into your blood. Your large intestine is where most of your gut bacteria should be in order to break down your food and excrete the waste. Having SIBO means that the bacteria residing in your large intestine have overgrown and are now growing in places they shouldn't be.

Two years ago I planted raspberries and blackberries in my back yard, right under my living room window. At first they both grew simultaneously, but one morning I came outside and the blackberries seemed to have doubled in size overnight. Over the next few months this plant grew like a weed. It took over the entire planter box and began covering my window. I pruned it, but despite my best efforts shoots soon began to grow up everywhere, including in my lawn. We decided to pull the plant out entirely, but for the last two years I have still had to contend with blackberry shoots growing in places they do not belong.

In a person with SIBO, bacteria levels in the small intestine rise and interfere with the normal absorption process. If your small intestine has trouble absorbing the nutrients it needs, this can have a detrimental effect on the rest of your body. It can damage the lining of your stomach or even lead to serious vitamin and iron deficiencies.

While there are various causes for SIBO, it often occurs in people who struggle with candida overgrowth and whose diet is high in sugary or starchy foods, such as bread or pasta. The bacteria ferment these sugars, causing gas emission and bloating.

The symptoms are similar to those of irritable bowel syndrome and other gastrointestinal disorders. In fact, SIBO is increasingly being researched as a possible cause of IBS. Symptoms include: bloating, diarrhea, nausea, vomiting, malnutrition, fatigue, asthma, joint pain, and weight loss. It can also lead to skin conditions such as rashes, acne, psoriasis, eczema, and rosacea, as well as mental health conditions such as depression.

SIBO, parasites, and yeast overgrowth are all the result of an infection in the gut. One or all three may be contributing to your symptoms, but SIBO is treatable, and by making some basic lifestyle changes, most notably to your diet, you'll be able to bring back the balance to your gut.

Recommended treatment

You can arm yourself with the foods you need for total health, for instance through the Autoimmune Protocol (AIP) low-FODMAP diet. This will help you decrease inflammation, alkalize your body, lower your blood glucose levels, and eliminate toxins, while also giving you the nutrients your body needs. Once your body is balanced you can simply follow a clean diet. You can read more about clean eating in the next section, and if you feel inspired to make some diet changes you could try following my five-day meal plan (see p. 141).

High-quality, natural supplements can also help to restore your body's natural balance. In addition to the supplements I list when discussing gut repair, I also used Microb-Clear supplied by Dr. Amy Myers, M.D. This blend of powerful botanicals is available on her website and may help to improve your symptoms. You will also need to take a high-quality probiotic (Dr. Myers' Primal Earth Probiotic is specifically designed not to feed certain strains of good bacteria, which is critical in treating SIBO). Finally, after a couple of weeks of following this protocol you will want to rotate through antimicrobial supplements such as oil of oregano, black seed oil, or grapefruit seed extract to kill off additional microbes.

Candida overgrowth

Candida overgrowth was an enormous problem for me. It began when I was seventeen and clueless. My gut health problems started in high school with my first yeast infection, and continued until I was forty. I did not make the connection between my diet and the balance that was needed in my microbiome (community of bacteria) to keep me healthy and free of chronic yeast infections until more than two decades had passed. I would blame the healthcare system for this, but they were not responsible for my very real and serious addiction to sugar. That fell solely on me.

If you've never heard of candida, you may be surprised to learn that it's already present in your body. It's a form of yeast that lives in minimal amounts inside your mouth and intestines. It helps your body digest food and absorb the nutrients you need to survive.

The problem with candida occurs when it is overproduced. In the 'right' conditions there is no limit to how far it will spread through your body. If your body contains too much yeast you are putting yourself at risk of a host of health problems. The imbalance between good and bad bacteria can cause organ and tissue damage, and may eventually become a chronic condition. If your diet consists mostly of refined carbohydrates and sugar, you're putting yourself at risk. The same goes for alcohol. These items fuel the growth of yeast to beyond the healthy limit. The good news is that by recognizing the cause and symptoms you can start to treat the infection and get your life back on track.

In addition to diet, several other factors can contribute to a candida overgrowth. Since it's the healthy bacteria that help to keep candida levels in check, taking antibiotics reduces your natural defense mechanism. Oral contraceptives can also lead to candida overgrowth. Birth control pills increase our estrogen levels, which can raise our susceptibility to yeast. People who use corticosteroid inhalants to treat asthma are also at risk, and should follow hygiene guidance when cleaning their inhalers. In addition, steroids can weaken the body's immune system, making it easier for yeast to grow. In fact, anything that weakens your natural immune defense will increase your odds of contracting a yeast infection.

Finally, more serious diseases such as cancer and diabetes may cause candida infections. In a similar way to antibiotics, chemotherapy in cancer patients can kill off the healthy bacteria needed to prevent yeast overgrowth. Meanwhile, high levels of sugar in the mouths and other membranes of those with diabetes can become a fertile breeding ground for candida.

The symptoms of a candida infection vary from person to person. They may include any of the following:

1. **Skin and nail fungal infections.** Candida can lead to athlete's foot, ringworm, and toenail fungus, among other infections.
2. **Exhaustion.** If you constantly feel tired no matter how long you sleep, and it's a feeling that has lasted at least six months, candida may be to blame.
3. **Digestive issues.** Bloating, diarrhea, and constipation are common symptoms of candida.
4. **Mood disorders.** Candida can result in irritability, anxiety, depression, and mood swings.
5. **Vaginal and urinary tract infections.** Vaginal yeast and urinary tract infections can be caused by an overgrowth of candida.
6. **Thrush.** This yeast infection, which can appear in your mouth, vagina, or other parts of your body, provides an itchy and sore indication of candida.
7. **Focus issues.** Candida can leave you feeling unfocused, making it difficult to concentrate and remember things. It can also give a feeling of brain fog.
8. **Hormone changes.** If you notice that your hormone levels are less balanced than usual, for instance in the form of early menopause or lower sex drive, this could relate to a candida overgrowth.
9. **Interstitial cystitis.** IC flare-ups can also be brought on by excess yeast levels.

Recommended treatment

The first step to reducing your candida overload is to cut your natural sugar intake. Focus on following the candida diet, which avoids all refined sugars. You can also enhance your diet with natural supplements that will help to restore your body's balance. ProBiome's Candida Combat (available via Dr. Axe's website) is my personal go-to because it contains a blend of antioxidants, enzymes, prebiotics, and probiotics that help to support healthy yeast management. Finally, a high-quality coconut oil applied topically can act as a great antifungal treatment.

IBS

Irritable bowel syndrome is pretty common, yet I find most people who have it do not even realize it. In fact, estimates suggest that IBS affects anywhere from thirty-eight to ninety-six million Americans. Of those, only around six per cent have ever been diagnosed.

If you are frequently experiencing alternating bouts of diarrhea and constipation, as well as flatulence, changes in bowel movements or the appearance of your stool, acid reflux, nausea, bloating, or other problems in and around your abdominal area on a regular basis, you could be suffering from IBS.

For these symptoms to be categorized as IBS they would usually last for roughly three to six months, and symptoms would stick around for at least three consecutive days each month. Because it isn't a single disease that stems from a single cause, IBS can be difficult to diagnose and treat. Understanding the underlying causes of your symptoms will enable you to find the treatment path that works best for you.

Relief from symptoms is often experienced once normal bowel movements have resumed. What's normal for you may not be normal for someone else, but in general bowel movements should occur somewhere between three times a day and three times a week. Stool should pass fairly easily. It should have the texture of peanut butter and be around the size of a sausage. Normal stool is usually brown or golden brown in color. Anything that drastically varies from this could point to bowel problems or IBS.

If you're suffering from IBS, the enzymes, muscles, and nerves in your digestive tract are not functioning normally. However, different factors may be responsible for different symptoms in each person. Some people may have multiple causes that need to be addressed, ranging from leaky gut to small intestinal bacterial or yeast overgrowth. Other causes may include parasites, food allergies or sensitivities, and stress.

Recommended treatment
The way IBS symptoms are eliminated depends on the root cause, but there are steps you can take to keep digestive problems to a minimum. Start by cutting out anything in your diet that could be damaging your gut, especially inflammatory substances such as gluten, sugar, soy, alcohol, and caffeine. Load up on the acids and enzymes your body needs to properly digest your food. Take a probiotic supplement to maintain healthy levels of bacteria in your gut. You can also take supplements such as collagen or L-glutamine, and of course, maintain healthy levels of

vitamins A, C, E, omega-3, and zinc. It's also critical to stay as stress-free as possible, so keep enjoying the activities you love most.

Stress, anxiety, and depression

Are you suffering from depression? When you get stressed out or anxious do you have to contend with an almost immediate flare-up of IC symptoms? Stress, anxiety, and depression are normal feelings that many people experience from time to time (though some with greater severity than others), but when this affects your quality of life it may be time to dig a little deeper. There are a number of ways to manage your stress, which we will discuss in Chapter 9, but when it comes to chronic stress, anxiety, and depression one of the major underlying causes may be related to leaky gut.

This is because gut health affects our serotonin, a chemical neurotransmitter responsible for maintaining mood balance. Serotonin is produced in the brain and in the intestines; in fact, eighty percent of serotonin is produced in the gut. When leaky gut is in play it can cause a serotonin deficiency, which causes inflammation and affects mood. The problem here is that chronic inflammation in the brain is difficult to recognize because our brains do not have pain receptors. However, research has shown that patients with depression typically display inflammation markers.

The connection between the brain and our intestines comes via the vagus nerve, which connects them. We feel this gut-brain link when we are too nervous to eat, or when we are stressed to the point that we have digestive issues. Managing symptoms is certainly important, but reducing inflammation by addressing its root cause will help in managing emotions that may get the best of us at times.

The reason this neurotransmitter is important is that it not only carries signals along and between nerves, but influences the majority of our brain cells. As well as being linked to mood it can impact bowel function, clotting, sleep, appetite, digestion, nausea, bone density, and sexual function. As serotonin levels affect our mood – specifically in terms of depression and anxiety – it seems critical to ensure that gut health is a core focus when attempting to address these symptoms.

Recommended treatment

Repairing leaky gut is crucial as this will affect serotonin levels. Dr.

Myers' NeuroCalm Mag powder relieves stress, anxiety, and depression by regulating serotonin levels, which may help you feel calmer and more relaxed, while also improving mental health and cognitive function. I would also recommend Kavinace from NeuroScience, which promotes sleep as well as alleviating stress and anxiety.

*

By this point the importance of maintaining a healthy gut should be clear. The functions of the gut are so vast it makes perfect sense that the largest part of the immune system is located there. Chronic inflammation is widely believed to be the root cause of most disease, which means that gut health should be one of our primary focuses when addressing a number of health concerns. If you have any of the symptoms mentioned in this chapter it may be necessary to have a Comprehensive Digestive Stool Analysis (CDSA) done, and possibly also a SIBO breath test, which will serve to identify GI disorders.

People often state how unfair it is that they suffer with IC, and I agree. It is unfair. Yet, in this day and age I believe we are all at risk of chronic inflammation, and though not everyone is suffering from IC, many are dealing with health issues of their own. Our modern lifestyle seems almost entirely incongruent with our genetic makeup. Our bodies are under continual strain from our diet, which is made up of foods that our bodies can no longer tolerate or even recognize. Added to this, we are afflicted by a heavy toxic burden caused by the environment we live in and, for many of us, the sedentary lifestyles we lead.

Building a healthy microbiome

One of the most important ways to maintain gut integrity is to focus on a healthy microbiome. According to Amy Myers, author of *The Autoimmune Solution*, we need more "friendly" bacteria. She writes: "The friendly bacteria that live in the gut are incredibly helpful. They make it possible for you to digest your food, and they maintain the lining of your intestinal walls, the epithelium."

The gut relies on trillions of bacteria that live within the intestines. In fact, we possess ten times more microbial cells than human cells. You probably don't even realize it, but you're carrying around a good few pounds' worth of microbes – including fungi, viruses, and bacteria – in your intestines, and all these symbiotic microbial cells cause us to become sick if they get out of balance (known as "dysbiosis").

Comprising 100 trillion organisms in total, the microbiome in the gut provides an incredibly diverse ecosystem. This ecosystem is affected by diet, chronic stress, infections, antibiotics, and toxins, including environmental toxins. Additionally, gut flora (microbiota) plays a role in the gut-brain axis, which, as we saw above, links the gastrointestinal tract and central nervous system. Since the gut contains the highest quantity of bacteria, as well as the greatest number of species in comparison with the rest of the body, gut flora provides a vital barrier against pathogenic organisms.

Focusing on gut microbiota (microorganisms), which are responsible for breaking down and absorbing nutrients, is extremely important when addressing IC. Maintaining healthy, balanced gut microbiota is crucial, since this ecosystem is directly linked to the health of our immune systems. However, it is worth noting that the human microbiome is made up of communities of symbiotic bacteria that inhabit various regions of the body, including our skin, mouth, eyes, genitals, and intestines. The focus must always be on our overall health as we strive to maintain balance within the body as a whole. To give you an example, focusing solely on your gut health without maintaining your mouth's oral microbiota will allow opportunistic microbes or pathogens to become out of control, and since the mouth's microbiota is connected to the lungs' microbiota, one will affect the other. The microbiome is responsible for a number of functions, none of which should be minimized since each plays an important part in our overall health and well-being.

A decrease in friendly gut bacteria will allow pathogens to get out of control, and an infection involving one or more can allow SIBO, yeast overgrowth, and parasites to set in. These gut infections will contribute to leaky gut, pushing us further up the autoimmune spectrum. Pathogens can coexist in our microbiome and may, in fact, be beneficial, but if these opportunistic, disease-causing microbes get out of hand they will disrupt the good bacteria. Our future health depends on the microbiome, which is made up of some 10,000 different microbial species, which maintain its diversity. An imbalance here will affect your health!

Mast cell activation
As we have already established, a range of factors can damage the

intestinal and bladder linings, including certain foods, drugs, toxins, and stress. These can contribute to the activation of mast cells. Located throughout the body – in our connective tissue, under the surface of the skin, in the bladder, the respiratory system, and the digestive and urinary tracts – they essentially mediate our system's inflammation. They are necessary and critical to our survival. Mast cells are our first line of defense against infections, helping our bodies heal and protect themselves from various pathogens.

Nevertheless, when mast cells become overactive they can cause chronic inflammation. That is because they store neurotransmitters – chemical messengers, like histamine and interleukins – that can cause inflammation or allergic reactions by way of damage to mucous membranes and tissue, or in the widening of blood vessels. Mast cells can be the trigger for anything from asthma and eczema to conjunctivitis, autoimmune diseases, and reproductive disorders.

When mast cells in the bladder lining become stimulated from urine that is either too acidic or toxic they begin to secrete the content of their granules. This can cause significant inflammation in the bladder. An autoimmune response is often triggered, and the lining of the bladder begins to leak as it becomes increasingly permeable.

This is where it becomes important to understand that the microbiome community in the bladder must remain balanced for your bladder to remain healthy. If there is imbalance among the bacteria, archaea, viruses, and fungi in your urine you may find yourself at greater risk of bladder dysfunction, including leaks in the bladder lining and other health issues. There is also a correlation between the bacteria in your intestines and mast cell activation in your bladder. Furthermore, studies are currently examining the relationship between bacteria in the urine and vagina, especially given that so many people who suffer from interstitial cystitis also suffer from vaginitis.

Functional medicine relates the root cause of most chronic illnesses to inflammation, leaky gut, toxicity, stress, and food sensitivity. Dr. Amy Myers proposes an autoimmune spectrum, where patients rank themselves depending on their symptoms. This is a useful model, in that minor symptoms left unchecked can lead to chronic conditions, including autoimmune disorders. It can also help to explain why so many people who suffer from interstitial cystitis also suffer from allergies, chronic fatigue, fibromyalgia, and a host of other autoimmune conditions.

Whether we are high or low on the spectrum we must listen to our bodies. They are telling us they need better care and attention. In order to restore balance and decrease inflammation, our bodies need proper nourishment and protection. This is the only way to restore the bladder's diverse microbiome, which will in turn protect against infection, damage, and disease, and will also serve to reduce the symptoms of interstitial cystitis. We must always attempt to address the root cause of a problem rather than the symptoms alone. This includes examining your diet, finding better coping mechanisms for stress in your life, healing leaky gut, supporting liver function, and reducing the level of toxins to which your body is exposed.

*

How much time have you spent looking back over your life and writing down all the little signs that emerged before you were diagnosed with IC? Mapping this out will help you and your doctor understand where things began to go wrong, and what laid the foundation for it to develop. Most importantly, it will give you both a clear picture of what needs to be addressed so you can restore balance to your body.

I grew up in a fairly health-conscious home. My parents exercised regularly, and we ate a healthier diet than most families. When I hit middle-school age I developed chronic sinus infections, which were of course treated with antibiotics. In ninth grade I began having random dizzy spells, which would leave me unable to stand. This was not diagnosed as Ménière's disease until I was in my mid-twenties. The high school years were unkind. I struggled with acne that would, as I got older, turn into adult cystic acne (acne that causes cysts). I had my first yeast infection at seventeen and struggled with chronic yeast infections, which continued until the age of forty. As my sinus and allergy problems grew worse I began suffering from migraines whenever the weather (or even just the wind) changed. I also struggled with anxiety from a young age, and it grew worse as I got older.

My sinus infections eventually morphed into daily congestion and my nose always felt blocked, which reduced the oxygen flow to my brain. This made me feel tired and I struggled to focus. In order to stay on my feet and functioning I began taking 800 mg of Motrin (ibuprofen) plus Claritin-D 24 (a decongestant that contains pseudoephedrine) every day for many years. Despite pleading with various doctors and specialists to push through my request to have my deviated septum repaired and my nasal airways opened up so I could breathe properly, I was assured that the quantity I was taking was perfectly safe and that I did not need surgery. Around the same time I began dealing with regular nausea and constipation, but foolishly assumed this was normal.

Then, at the age of twenty-four, we went through a very difficult season as a family. The stress took a physical toll on me, leaving me so drained that it was a struggle just to keep my head above water. Between the stress, the migraines, the sinus infections, the dizzy spells, the recurring yeast infections, and finally a UTI (treated with antibiotics), I was fed up and decided I wanted to come off all these medications so my body could rest. I found a supplement to help minimize the occurrence of yeast infections, reduced my sodium intake to address the Ménière's, and Tom and I saved up so I could afford to have the nasal surgery.

In August 2005 – after the surgery, another round of antibiotics, and six weeks of healing – I could finally breathe! The regular migraines went away immediately, and I no longer needed the Motrin or the Claritin-D 24. I thought I was free and clear, but that January I was diagnosed with interstitial cystitis. As the years passed I developed several food intolerances, brain fog, eczema, adrenal fatigue, hormone imbalance, and digestive issues. I continued to struggle with acne and recurring yeast infections, frequent colds, allergies, sporadic migraines due to stress, and lower back pain that was debilitating at times.

I'm sharing all of this with you because until I really looked at what had been going on it was all a bit of a guessing game. Years of treating just about every issue with antibiotics, pumping toxic chemicals into my body, and poor diet led to a compromised immune system, leaky gut, poor liver function, toxicity, infections, and IC. Roadmapping it helped me understand what had gone wrong, but it also allowed me to roadmap my way out so I could get my health and life back!

This morning before work Tom and I, who are now empty nesters and grandparents, started our day with a five-mile bike ride. We took a path that led us down a hill; the same hill I started walking when I first decided to get in shape some eight years ago. I smiled as I glided down that hill and past our old home because I never thought I would be where I am today. I can't help but feel excited about what lies ahead, and I am blessed to have this opportunity to share my journey with you.

A couple of years ago I read a study on IC which concluded that for those with severe symptoms the pain is comparable to stage four renal cancer. What an enormous burden to carry! I believe that "IC warrior" seems a fitting title for each and every one of us. As I look back on the last thirteen years of my life I cannot believe I have come so far. Every day feels like a gift, and I have more energy, clarity, mental focus, and physical stamina than I have had in my entire life. You can also have all this, so let's get into some specifics.

Steps to repairing leaky gut

First and foremost, you must change your diet! You have to remove inflammatory foods and begin eating foods that are nutrient-rich and high in fiber, which will give your digestive tract a break from hard-to-digest foods. Here is a simple test: if you do not recognize the ingredients on the labels, the chances are your body will not recognize them either. Second, begin taking high-quality supplements that will aid in gut repair and work to diversify your microbiome. As always, use the recommended doses of any supplements you use, and talk it through with your healthcare provider first.

Here are my top tips:

1. Consume only bone broth for two to three days if tolerable. If you can only do the broth by itself for one day that's fine, just add some squash and spinach to it after that, and protein if you feel you need it. The ideal solution would be to drink the broth for up to five days so your digestive tract can rest. Bone broth contains amino acids, minerals, and collagen, all of which will promote a healthy gut. Make sure you use a high-quality, organic bone broth. I personally love Pressery bone broth from Costco, but there are plenty out there to choose from. Better yet, make your own! I always have some in the fridge and often drink a warm cup between lunch and dinner. I also take every opportunity to cook with bone broth, adding it to most of my recipes.

2. Take hydrolyzed collagen powder once or twice per day. Adding this powdered connective tissue from cows and fish to your coffee, smoothies, oatmeal, or juice can really help. Not only does it deliver a high concentration of protein; it also helps to improve gut and bone health, soothes achy joints, and reduces the appearance of wrinkles. Collagen contains amino acids, specifically glycine, and is a key structural protein. It is one of the body's most important building blocks and strengthens our connective tissues, including skin, tendons, ligaments, bones, and cartilage.

3. Use probiotics to diversify your microbiome. Probiotics are the bacteria in your gut that line your digestive tract and support your body's ability to absorb nutrients and fight infection, but sometimes they need a bit of a boost. These live bacteria and yeasts help to support immune system and healthy digestion. You should already be using them, but if not start immediately and take them daily. Make sure it is a high-quality supplement, containing a minimum of fifty billion CFUs of live cultures, NutraFlora fiber, vegetarian capsules, and at least twelve strains of bacteria. There are different types of probiotics to address specific gut issues, and rotating brands is wise. It is best to take your probiotics with a meal that contains prebiotics because prebiotics act as food for probiotics.

4. Consume prebiotics. Prebiotics are soluble fibers that change the composition and activity of your microbiota and stimulate the growth of good bacteria in the body. Foods containing prebiotics include leeks, onions, garlic, asparagus, bananas, tomatoes, berries, and flaxseed. Prebiotics are living organisms, and they need to stay alive so they can grow in your gut, providing food for probiotics. Avoid prebiotics if you are suffering with SIBO or candida.

5. Use digestive enzyme supplements. Take one or two capsules before each meal as they aid digestion and will help you derive more nutrition from your food. Leaky gut stops us from absorbing what we should from our food, so these supplements will help redress the balance.

6. Take betaine and pepsin supplements. This will support your stomach acid in breaking down protein so that it can be predigested. You could take one or more capsules before each meal.

7. Add immunoglobulin G (IgG) supplements to your routine. This will help boost your immune system, aiding gut repair and microbial balance.

8. Take omega-3 fish oil. This helps to manage immune function, connective tissue, and inflammatory response. Dr. Deckert recommends a triglyceride (TG) of omega-3, which is the most natural and potent form, making it preferable to ethyl ester (EE) fish oils. It also has a longer shelf life. Take between one and four capsules per day.

9. Try taking acetyl-glutathione. This form of glutathione is absorbed more effectively than other forms as it remains more stable through the digestive tract. It provides intracellular antioxidant support and healthy cell function, supporting detoxification, immune response, and amino acid transport across cell membranes.

10. Use L-glutamine powder. This amino acid is the most prevalent amino acid in the bloodstream. It aids cells in lining the intestines and is involved in more metabolic processes than any other amino acid. Capable of passing through the blood-brain barrier, it also promotes mental alertness, improving memory and enhancing mood. It assists in digestion and muscle growth, fights cancer, and helps to regulate blood sugar levels. L-glutamine powder is a vital nutrient for rebuilding and repairing the intestines. It helps in combating leaky gut, balances mucus production (which improves IBS symptoms), supports detoxification and immune function, and repairs tissue.

11. Take liver support capsules. Your liver is one of the hardest-working organs in your body. It is constantly working to filter toxins out of your bloodstream, and is responsible for regulating blood sugar levels, creating bile, producing cholesterol, and much more. This supplement offers your liver the support it needs for optimal function, detoxification, and bile production, while helping to protect liver cells.

12. Buy zinc carnosine. This artificially produced carnosine derivative is believed to be three times more effective as a compound than as individual ingredients. It protects the gastrointestinal system and helps to repair the gut. It can be used to treat indigestion, gastritis and gastric ulcers, and dyspepsia. Zinc carnosine supports liver health, promotes nutrient absorption, reduces inflammation, and boosts immunity.

13. Take Vitamin D and Vitamin A supplements. It's worth checking with your doctor first to find out if you have any vitamin deficiencies. Vitamin D is important for overall health and supports the immune system, as well as brain and bone health. If you have a deficiency, try taking a D3-K2 supplement. Vitamin A is an antioxidant that fights free radicals in the body, reducing inflammation. It also supports immune function. (Please note that vitamin A supplements should be avoided in pregnancy.)

14. Eat whole foods that are rich in probiotics, fiber, and healthy fats. (Follow the food list in the next chapter for further guidance.) To foster a healthy and diverse microbiome, eat a variety of fruits and vegetables from good, nutrient-rich soil.

15. Eat fermented foods. Fermented foods contain live microorganisms that flourish once they reach our digestive tract. Fermented foods include kombucha (fermented tea), miso (fermented soybeans), kefir (organic, fermented goat or sheep milk), sauerkraut (fermented cabbage), and kimchi (fermented vegetables). Avoid fermented foods if you are suffering with SIBO or candida.

16. Try intermittent fasting. Leave twelve to sixteen hours of fasting between dinner and breakfast to allow your digestive tract to rest. This could be done every day or two to three times per week.

17. Get outside. In a continued effort to strengthen the immune system, you must work to increase your microbial exposure. Put the antibacterial hand sanitizers away and get outside! Gardening is an excellent way to expose your immune system to the trillions of microbes in the soil. Go for a hike and get some fresh air. Our immune systems depend on exposure to both good and bad organisms, otherwise they get out of whack and are thrown off balance. We need more exposure to the variety of microorganisms that usually populate the body. The human microbiota is shaped by our diet, lifestyle, and microbial exposure to the environment, and this is absolutely necessary for human health. It is not harmful to expose our bodies to bacteria, fungi, archaea, viruses, and other pathogens; in fact, most are beneficial.

18. Drink plenty of water. One of the best ways to address leaky gut syndrome is to drink plenty of water. Bowel problems can lead to chronic dehydration, which will cause your waste matter to harden and stagnate. As a result, the bacteria in the stool inflame the intestinal lining. The experts recommend a minimum water intake of three liters a day! It's also worth cutting out caffeine, alcohol, and sugar-filled drinks, which can exacerbate intestinal issues. Make sure you are drinking filtered or distilled water, which will minimize exposure to toxins.

Additional supplements or nutrients you may wish to add in to aid with gut repair include: licorice root (if tolerable), quercetin, marshmallow root, slippery elm, caprylic acid, and Candisol.

It can take anywhere from one to six months to heal leaky gut, but you should start to feel better fairly quickly. Don't take all these supplements at once because too much of a good thing – even high-quality supplements – can put too much strain on the liver. Talk with your doctor about which ones you should be taking and in what quantity.

Do you really want your health back? What physical limitations are holding you back, and what would you be prepared to give up to remove them? I'm not going to lie; removing trigger foods such as gluten, dairy, soy, sugar, and GMOs is a big deal. And drinking bone broth for a few days may sound dreadful, but it's not impossible. You have been down long enough. It's time to get to work. It's time to take control. It's time to get your life back! Now is your time.

Chapter 7

WHAT YOU ARE EATING MATTERS

"The way to get started is to quit talking and begin doing."

Animator and film director Walt Disney

We know this is true, yet often we ignore the wisdom that tells us to make sensible choices when it comes to our food. Our flesh always wants more. It is never satisfied, and it constantly screams at us, tempting us to give in to its many desires and cravings. Unfortunately, what the body most often craves is sugar, carbs, dairy, and junk! When we are young we can often get away with eating pizza and drinking soda as if these are the only forms of food on the planet. This is partly because our bodies are new and strong, and our metabolisms are faster. But then our twenties hit, and we realize that, not only has this stopped being the case, but it never really was. We thought we were invincible, and that our parents' incessant nagging about the benefits of vegetables was more of a suggestion than actual wisdom.

It turns out that what we eat will make or break us when it comes to our health. For those of us who suffer from IC, diet plays a far larger role with regard to our overall health than we may understand. We need to take a closer look at the foods we are consuming to better comprehend the direct benefits that will come from implementing a strategic diet. Diet can both cause and contribute to chronic inflammation, which is dangerous and can damage the body if left unchecked, and is believed to play a part in a number of illnesses. The foods we choose to eat can either increase inflammation in the bladder and irritate it further, or decrease inflammation, providing the bladder with an opportunity to heal. Foods that have been deemed inflammatory should be avoided at all costs!

It's worth noting here that some people claim to have healed themselves of IC by simply changing their diet and eating mostly vegetables, with alkalization being their primary focus. Those of us who suffer from severe IC may be tempted to protest loudly, but let's think about this for just a moment. First of all, we know that there are varying degrees of IC. We also know that if an individual possesses certain genetic variants, or if there are underlying gut issues, the body will struggle to digest and absorb nutrients from food, further increasing our vulnerability to toxic buildup. We are aware that additional health issues vary from person to person, and understand that IC is multifactorial. Finally, it's clear that some people have been misdiagnosed with IC.

Taking all this into consideration, it may be possible that a diet change is enough to help some people rid themselves of IC. However, making this a blanket statement is misleading. If you are like me, you will have already tried this and know that it doesn't work, which is why you get worked up at the mere mention of such a claim. However, eating a healthy diet in conjunction with proper supplementation, while simultaneously reducing your toxic burden and working to heal your gut, will bring support and balance to your body. Your diet is an essential foundation that must be laid properly for good health to flourish.

Most of the foods, beverages, and products we use on our skin contain toxins in the form of chemicals and additives. We must understand that toxic buildup is making us sick! We need to acknowledge that things like preservatives, artificial additives, and GMOs are man-made, and the extent to which we are currently consuming them is having a direct effect on our overall health. Eating cleanly while decreasing your toxic burden and maintaining a healthy microbiome will offer your body the support it needs to detox itself, ridding the cells of toxic buildup while increasing its ability to absorb the nutrients it needs from proper foods. This will allow the cells to repair themselves and assist in the body's overall healing, reducing inflammation and restoring balance. The body's cells are the backbone of our physiology, which means that healthy cells equal a healthy body.

Americans are assaulted day in, day out with an onslaught of chemicals, producing a toxic burden we were not physically designed to withstand, and slowly poisoning us. Billions of pounds of toxic chemicals are released into the environment, and federal officials have deemed many of these hazardous to our health. To further add to the chemical assault, 2,000 new chemicals enter the environment each year in the U.S., and many lack the substantial testing needed to determine their impact on our health weighed against levels of exposure. A report from the National Toxicology Program said: "Many of the products that you consume contain detectable traces of chemicals in them while the government maintains minimal involvement in setting chemical regulations which are needed to keep consumers safe."

We need to be really careful about the foods we are consuming. In 2016, Organic Authority published an article based on the findings of the Environmental Working Group (EWG), which alerted consumers that billions of gallons of recycled wastewater from oil and gas drilling facilities had been used in irrigating crops within California's Central Valley. This is even more worrying given the fact that, in the last three years, oil companies have admitted to using twenty million pounds of chemicals containing numerous toxins and unidentifiable chemical ingredients. Of the two tests conducted to determine whether or not toxic chemicals were safe for use in crop irrigation, neither soil samples nor root vegetables were analyzed for their potential health risks.

I don't know about you, but I take little solace from knowing that the crops filling the produce section of my local grocery store have been grown in lightly treated wastewater derived from oil fields. It is unfortunate that we live in a day and age in which we are bombarded by toxins from every angle. However, while we cannot change the ways of the world overnight, we can take responsibility for our health by paying attention to what is going on around us. We have a collective voice, and if we choose to use it and direct it toward government agencies we can help to bring about change, demanding that safety measures which protect the public and the environment are put in place. You also have a private vote. You vote every time you choose to pull out your hard-earned cash to buy something.

We are the "generation of now." We want everything right away, and the idea that "patience is a virtue" seems to be lost on most of us. Our impatience has led to the pursuit of instant gratification, specifically regarding what we eat, as convenience dominates the culture. Somewhere along the way we officially adopted the Burger King slogan, "Have it Your Way," and made it our national motto. The American diet leaves little to be desired, with processed and packaged foods providing quick options, while "portion distortion" has evolved into the new norm.

For those who are convinced that there is no real proof that we are, as a whole, affected by the current toxicity in our food, let's take a closer look. Child obesity has doubled in the past three decades; quadrupling in teens. Fifty percent of women in the United States will develop cancer in their lifetime, as will one-third of men, accounting for one in four deaths.

Nearly thirty-one million Americans have high cholesterol, putting them at risk of heart disease and stroke. Heart disease is currently the leading cause of death in the U.S. Due to livestock being treated with antibiotics, human resistance to antibiotics has skyrocketed, resulting in 23,000 U.S. deaths each year, due in large part to our consumption of animals and animal products.

Think back to elementary school for a moment. How many of your classmates were obese? How many struggled to sit still and focus in class? How many had peanut allergies, or were intolerant to gluten or dairy? Do you remember hearing about IBS or celiac disease (instances of which have increased by 500 percent) in grade school? Peanut allergies have risen by a whopping 300 percent in the last thirty years. The fact is, the ingredients in the foods we consume are bad for our bodies. We desperately need to eat fiber, naturally occurring vitamins, moderate amounts of high-quality protein, antioxidants, minerals, and healthy amounts of fat, sodium, and unrefined sugar in order to run at full capacity. Avoiding foods that contain carcinogens, synthetic chemicals, artificial colors, sweeteners, trans fats, and GMOs is an absolute must if you want to get healthy. Processed and packaged foods are toxic. They have been linked to a number of health issues, including diabetes, high cholesterol, heart disease, cancer, chronic fatigue, mood swings, obesity, diabetes, chronic inflammation, and a host of other things.

Let's stop pretending that we can't see the ill effects of our poor diet as a nation. Let's quit putting our "busy" schedules ahead of our own health and the health of our children. Let's check our laziness at the door and begin to take control of our health. It's time to give attention and priority to what we are taking in, and to begin to make wise choices that will lead to healthier lifestyles. We reap what we sow, and if we sow bad seeds in terms of our eating habits we should not be surprised by the weeds (weight and health issues) that are growing up all around us, choking the life out of us.

I should probably state here that I categorically do not believe in dieting! That's because dieting is temporary, as are the results. We usually become more aware of the fact that we have not been eating properly and need to commit to doing better around Christmas, New Year's Eve, summer holidays, and other major events, such as weddings or high school reunions. All of a sudden we pull out the scales and hop on, only to be shocked by what we see when we look down between our feet. We plunge ourselves into eating more fruits and vegetables, while cutting back on sugar and carbs. We recommit to exercise, saunas, and seaweed wraps in an effort to detoxify, burn calories, and lose those unwanted pounds. But dieting is temporary and often involves taking extreme measures. Some focus on a high-protein, low-carb, or low-calorie meals, while others involve a ridiculously extreme cleanse (such as watermelon for breakfast, lunch, and dinner). Don't make it about following a diet. Make eating healthily your lifestyle! This means that it becomes who you are rather than a quick fix, and you get to be that person year-round without the pressure of New Year's resolutions or swimsuit season. It is far better to be realistic and make wise choices every day than to get hyped up over the latest dieting craze that is sweeping the nation.

Focus should therefore be placed on making the right choices when selecting our foods, and not about the number we see when we hop on the scales. Put the scales away! I am huge fan of "eating clean" because the focus is on moderation. It's about eating foods that are free of chemicals, additives, and hormones, and that have not been processed or refined.

Eating clean simply means that your diet primarily consists of organic whole foods that are as close to their natural state as you can get them. Before you freak out and toss this book at the wall, let me give you some suggestions that are easy to pick up next time you are at the grocery store. These few changes will get you off to a great start as you begin the process of eating clean.

Clean eating food list
Bacon: organic, uncured. Brand: Applegate. Bacon is extremely unhealthy, so minimize consumption.
Beverages: kombucha, coconut kefir, herbal teas, raw vegetable juices.
Bread: sourdough (fermented) or Ezekiel bread (sprouted).
Butter: imported, raw butter, ghee. Brand: Kerrygold Pure Irish.
Canned goods: organic, BPA-free. Avoid if possible, opting for fresh ingredients instead.
Cheese: raw, imported, organic, from grass-fed animals. Feta (goat or sheep).
Chocolate: imported, organic, dark chocolate, minimum seventy percent cocoa.
Dairy: raw, organic, non-GMO, from 100 percent grass-fed animals, non-homogenized; coconut, organic almond, organic kefir, macadamia, cashew, sheep.

Deli meat: organic (nitrate, antibiotic, GMO, and hormone-free). Brand: Applegate. Turkey breast, roast chicken breast, roast beef.

Eggs: organic, free-range.

Fermented foods: sauerkraut, kefir, pickled cabbage, carrots, turnips, cucumbers, onions, kombucha, miso soup, kimchi, raw cheese.

Fish: fresh, wild-caught anchovies, catfish, flounder, salmon, trout, mackerel, ahi tuna.

Flour: (this can be tricky!) organic coconut flour, almond flour, quinoa flour, amaranth flour, einkorn flour, cassava flour, arrowroot flour.

Grains: organic quinoa, teff (a staple grain for Ethiopia), amaranth, chia seeds, wild rice (soak overnight and rinse before cooking), sprouted ancient grains.

Herbs: ginger, ginseng, cinnamon, turmeric, cayenne, parsley, licorice, yarrow, mint, marshmallow root, plantain.

Honey: organic, raw manuka honey.

Juice: organic, 100 percent vegetable, aloe vera, and pear juice are gentle on the bladder.

Legumes: lentils, anasazi beans, peas, black beans, garbanzo beans (soak for twelve to twenty-four hours beforehand, then rinse and cook).

Meat: organic, grass-fed beef, bison, chicken, duck, lamb, turkey, wild game.

Nuts: organic or raw chestnuts, cashews, almonds (soak for twelve to twenty-four hours beforehand).

Oats: certified gluten-free (in order to avoid cross-contamination), sprouted.

Oil: organic, cold-pressed, extra virgin olive, coconut, sesame, walnut, flaxseed, avocado, almond, macadamia.

Pasta: gluten-free, imported (or substitute with organic squash or zucchini spaghetti).

Popcorn: organic, air-popped.

Potatoes: organic white or sweet potatoes, yams.

Produce: fresh, organic, or wild.

Rice: organic wild or black rice (soak for twelve to twenty-four hours beforehand and rinse).

Salad dressing: organic olive oil with apple cider vinegar or balsamic, or a dash of lemon (if tolerable for your bladder).

Salt: unrefined French grey sea salt, kosher sea salt, or Himalayan pink salt.

Seeds: sprouted chia, flaxseed, pumpkin, hemp.

Snacks: organic, gluten-free; no preservatives, refined sugar, artificial flavors, or food coloring.

Soy sauce: organic, non-GMO, gluten-free tamari, or substitute with coconut aminos.

Squash: organic acorn, butternut, or pumpkin (you can make spaghetti from these).

Sweeteners: 100 percent maple syrup, coconut sugar, organic raw honey, Stevia, coconut nectar, monk fruit.

Tea: organic, loose-leaf marshmallow leaf and root, corn silk,chamomile, licorice, ginger, nettle-leaf (which contains antihistamines).

Tomatoes: (least acidic) yellow pear, Caro Rich, Georgia Streak.

Tortillas: organic, corn, non-GMO, sprouted.

Water: filtered, distilled mineral water (drink six to eight glasses per day).

Yogurt: cultured goat, sheep, almond, coconut.

Eating out

Look for places that have healthy options and stay away from fried foods. Luna Grill is a great option and carries organic ingredients. If I have to grab fast food I eat at In-N-Out Burger (Protein Style) or Chick-fil-A (grilled chicken).

Additional pointers

* Avoid soy milk and all products that contain soy (including soy-lectin) unless it is organic and non-GMO.
* Always look for the orange butterfly (denoting the Non-GMO Project) when purchasing non-GMO products.
* Avoid artificial food colorings and dyes.
* Minimize gluten-free alternatives, as they are often unhealthy.
* Avoid using your microwave whenever possible, but if you do always heat food in microwave-safe glass.
* Reduce protein intake to 40-60 grams per day (depending on your weight) in order to reduce acid overload.
* Avoid corn and products containing corn unless it is labeled organic and non-GMO.

As you can see, I switched out many of my food items for healthier and, where possible, organic options. I realize this is not possible for everyone as there may be monetary or availability restraints, but if you are able to switch out even a few I would encourage you to do so. You don't have to go to your cupboards today and throw everything away if you don't have the means to replace it all with high-quality foods. But the next time you run out of butter, seek to replace it with Kerrygold Irish butter, and so on.

*

As you begin to pay attention to what you are eating it becomes more difficult to choose processed junk food because you know that what's in that package is literally poison for your body. The mere thought should make you nauseous, which means you are becoming more knowledgeable and actively seeking a healthier lifestyle for yourself and those you love.

When we first made the switch it was hard on the family wallet, but I believed it was extremely important for our health, and that we would either pay for it then or pay for it later in medical bills. If you cannot afford to buy seasonal, organic produce, select produce that has been minimally treated with pesticides. The EWG's yearly Dirty Dozen List provides a guide that will keep you abreast of which fruits and vegetables are safe to eat, and which have been heavily contaminated by harmful pesticides and should therefore be avoided. In 2018, strawberries and apples topped the list as most contaminated due to detectable pesticide residue. In California, the strawberry capital of the U.S., our already depleted soil and crops are drenched in 300 pounds of pesticides per acre of farmed strawberries. Lest you be deceived, it cannot all be washed away in your kitchen sink. Try your best to veer away from toxic chemicals, even in low doses, as they harm your health and the environment.

I get as many organic products as I can from Costco, Sprouts, Thrive Market, the local farmers' market, or Whole Foods, but to be honest some items are simply too expensive or too difficult to track down. If you get good at purchasing fruits and vegetables in place of processed snacks and foods, and begin cooking and eating at home, you will find that there are ways to keep your family budget within a reasonable limit. One of the biggest adjustments may be leaving sandwiches or prepackaged foods behind and opting instead for fresh ingredients. If you pack a lunch for work, or make your child a lunch for school, this may be where you decide to compromise because the alternative is just too much work and the uphill battle simply isn't worth it.

But overall this is not a battle you want to lose, and eating clean provides you with the opportunity to be creative. Taking leftovers for lunch, making a beautiful salad, or creating your own "lunchables" are great alternatives, and the options are limitless. Teaching our kids to eat healthily by setting a positive example is important for their minds and bodies, and as parents this is not an area in which we can afford to compromise. It's just too important.

When we begin eating more vegetables and fruits our palates may require a little time to adjust to the new flavors and textures, but just because something tastes different doesn't mean it is bad, and we should resist the urge to eat only what immediately tastes good. Keep an open mind, stay focused on the benefits, and give yourself time to adjust. You will find that after a while your body begins to crave broccoli. The only line I have drawn is with wheatgrass. It tastes horrible, and I am not a cow or dog with stomach issues!

I started my babies out eating green beans and spinach, and though there were days as they grew older when they put up a fight I made sure I won by convincing them that vegetables were their friends. Today they will eat anything that is put in front of them. This doesn't mean they love everything they eat, but they understand the benefits of choosing wisely, and thus no vegetable is left uneaten. They are fun to go out and eat with, and they are a pleasure to travel with because meals are not a source of stress but an area of pure enjoyment. Their open-mindedness has rubbed off on me as well, and I have begun eating raw fish, which you would know is a huge feat if you knew me personally!

Lastly, don't focus on what you *can't* eat; rather, focus on what you *can*. I gave you a list of options that are healthier for you, so fill your fridge and cupboard with these foods, which will offer you plenty of meal and snack options. Instead of pouting because you can't have that bag of Doritos, make a bowl of air-popped organic popcorn, drizzle a bit of raw butter over it, then sprinkle with Himalayan pink salt. You just need to be a little more creative.

As humans, we tend to veer away from any form of change since it pushes us out of our comfort zones and requires us to fight against our own will and desires. On some level we know that certain foods are bad for us and may irritate our bladders, but an unwillingness to compromise here and say no to inflammation-causing foods reveals a lack of wisdom. We convince ourselves that if we can keep flare-ups under control and at a tolerable minimum we can continue eating and drinking whatever we want. It's hard to break habits and fight against our cravings because it can make us uncomfortable, and it runs contrary to the philosophy that we should do whatever makes us happy. But this philosophy is an illusion that serves only to deceive us. Selfishness is really recklessness, as it often hurts not only ourselves but those we love. Indulging where we know we shouldn't may bring temporary happiness, but as the satisfaction wears off we are left to face the aftermath of our decisions. One of the best things we can do is choose our foods wisely so that we are healthy, strong, and able to care for our families while still making a point of enjoying life despite the dietary restrictions.

Beginning to focus on eating clean is a challenge, and it may be difficult for some, but most of us dealing with IC have grown accustomed to diet restraints. When I browse the diet food guides on the most popular IC websites my mind is boggled by the logic behind some of the recommendations. I believe that changing over to a clean diet is a major component in regaining our health, and therefore it should be instigated immediately. Drinking a vanilla milkshake to soothe a flare-up is helping no one; it's a cup full of chemicals, additives, and hormones. Put it down and walk away!

The pH factor

As we have already established, illness is most often caused by an imbalance in the body, so if we want to get well we need to re-establish this balance.

The body produces acid as a natural by-product of metabolism and is usually able to deal with it effectively. However, if you are exposed to toxins, have a poor diet, don't undertake regular exercise, and suffer from prolonged stress, your liver and kidneys may not be functioning properly, limiting their ability to get rid of acid. It is then stored in the spaces around the cells, causing acid buildup in the tissues. The blood becomes alkaline to compensate, and the body begins to work toward neutralizing the acid by stealing minerals (calcium, magnesium, potassium, and sodium) from vital organs and bones. Unfortunately, when the kidneys (metabolic acidosis) can no longer compensate for the excess acid that has accumulated it is no longer able to expel the acid from the body through urine, and the resulting fallout causes the blood to become acidic.

If you want your body to heal from chronic illness the pH balance of your blood needs to be restored to around 7.3. Keeping the right pH balance in the blood protects us against sickness and disease, while an imbalance will encourage fungus, bacteria, and viruses to breed and spread. So how can we cut acid levels in our bodies? As with other issues, diet plays a significant role. Did you know that eighty percent of the American diet is made up of acid-forming foods, with just twenty percent made up of alkalizing foods? When we eat acidic foods, or foods that create acid, blood flow to the bladder (among other parts of the body) is decreased. Mast cells are activated, releasing histamine and other inflammatory chemicals, which cause long-term inflammation along with further damage to cells and tissue.

Our goal throughout this book is to maintain balance, which we can do almost exclusively through making certain diet and lifestyle changes. An acid overload in the body must be neutralized by an intake of alkaline foods (see the foods I listed above) and by watching what we drink (cutting out alcohol, caffeine and citrus drinks, for example). The aim is to reach neutrality: when acid and alkaline levels are equal. This will depend on the choices we make each day.

Oxidative stress

Oxidative stress is caused by an increase of free radicals in the body due to toxins or poor nutrition. This results in an imbalance between the free radicals and antioxidants, which the body is unable to counter or detoxify. Harmful effects will soon ensue. Free radicals can damage our cells, leading to aging, disease, inflammation, and various disorders. Increasing your intake of natural antioxidants can assist in neutralizing free radicals, preventing cell damage, supporting detoxification, reducing inflammation, and restoring balance.

Start by increasing your intake of phytonutrient foods, which are rich in antioxidants. These include apples, artichokes, beets, blackberries, blueberries, broccoli, Brussels sprouts, cherries, cilantro, cinnamon, cumin, dark chocolate, kidney beans, oregano, plums, red grapes, spinach, kale, strawberries, melons, and turmeric. For added support in detoxification, you may want to consider glutathione supplements (see my earlier note about acetyl-glutathione on p. 73). Glutathione binds to free radicals and assists in eliminating toxins from the body, serving as its most significant detoxifier. Dr. Amy Myers sells a form called Acetyl-Glutathione (Citrisafe/Ovation) that allows for greater absorption, since it is not broken down in the gut. For more information visit the supplements section of her online store. Alternatively, N-Acetyl L-Cysteine (NAC) is an amino acid that is needed to make and replenish glutathione, and helps in the body's detoxification process. Available via integrativepro.com or on Amazon, this is a cheaper option.

Different types of food "allergy"

Certain foods trigger an autoimmune system response in some people. This can vary from a very dramatic reaction, where life is endangered, to a much subtler anatomical response, where antibodies are generated to fight the inflammation caused by a sensitivity to a particular food. Below are some of the antibodies that can cause an inflammatory response in the body:

- **Immunoglobulin G (IgG):** These antibodies have a slow inflammatory response. It can take up to three days before symptoms are felt, so it is more difficult to detect sensitivity or deficiency than it can be with other antibodies. Among other things, IgG antibodies are involved in the regulation of allergic reactions, so they can help to reduce reactions to inflammatory foods.

- **Immunoglobin A (IgA):** IgA is primarily found in the mucosal lining of the gut as well as in the urinary tract and vagina. These antibodies stop foreign invaders (parasites, viruses, and bacteria, including yeast overgrowth) from taking up residence. Depressed IgA levels will prevent you from getting the protection needed to ward off these invaders, so it's important that you find out if you are suffering from a deficiency.

- **Immunoglobin E (IgE):** These antibodies take immediate action on detecting a foreign intruder, creating an almost immediate immune response. The inflammatory response could be mild (hives) or life-threatening (anaphylaxis), for example in a peanut or bee sting allergy.

At the bare minimum, avoiding inflammatory (trigger) foods is necessary in healing the gut, and critical in reducing bladder inflammation. These foods should be removed from your diet immediately. You can figure out what your specific trigger foods are through an elimination diet, which will provide you with the clearest insight regarding the foods you are sensitive to.

Elimination diet

Begin by removing inflammatory foods, as well as any foods that were flagged in your immunoglobin test results. This will allow your metabolism to reset. Foods you are sensitive to are different from foods you are allergic to. Very few people (around one percent) are actually *allergic* to specific foods. When ingested, these foods create an almost immediate and very noticeable immune system (IgE) response in the body. Antibodies are instantly created to fight the invader. Symptoms may include severe skin reactions, anaphylaxis, chest pain, swelling of airways, shortness of breath, and serious digestive issues. In short, you will be in absolutely no doubt as to whether you have a genuine food allergy.

In contrast, those who have an IgG food sensitivity will have a slow or more delayed reaction, meaning that a response may not be noticeable for three to four days or even longer. The cause of your food intolerance could be an enzyme defect. Enzymes help to break down certain substances in food, and a lack of them will inhibit your body's ability to effectively break down and digest your food. Alternatively, it could be caused by toxins in the food, histamine buildup, leaky gut, or a hypersensitivity to food additives.

Having IC means that your bladder is damaged, and you will need to work hard to create an environment that allows healing to take place. But this will not happen unless you get serious about what you are eating and drinking, because consuming inflammatory foods or foods you are sensitive to will irritate your bladder, maintaining the chronic inflammation that puts you at risk of further damage while also laying the groundwork for autoimmunity. Understanding that food is medicine will dispel the common myths and misconceptions about food, for example, "There is no real proof that gluten or GMOs are bad for you."

You may be able to tolerate small quantities of certain foods once your gut has healed and bladder inflammation has subsided, and after you have pinpointed which are your trigger foods and removed them completely from your diet. But for right now, all focus should be placed on reducing bladder inflammation by avoiding these inflammatory foods for the next one to six months, depending on how you are feeling. From there, you can begin to reintroduce them one by one (except for gluten, conventional dairy, and GMOs, which should really be permanently avoided) every four days in order to gauge your body's response to them, allowing enough time for a delayed response to make itself known. Food sensitivity or intolerance can manifest in a number of ways, including skin issues (rashes, rosacea, hives, and acne), bladder irritation, digestive problems (stomach ache, IBS, bloating, and heartburn), migraines, asthma, brain fog, runny nose, an ongoing cough, a lethargic feeling, and headaches.

Unfortunately, the elimination of these foods alone will not be enough to stop some sufferers' bladder irritation. I hate to even go here, but please bear with me. I'm about to list two more categories that you may need to consider eliminating. So please resist the urge to throw this book down in utter frustration!

Foods that are high in oxalates

The diet you incorporate needs to be specific to you, and to your own unique genetic makeup. There is evidence to suggest foods that are high in oxalates (such as spinach, bran flakes, rhubarb, beets, potato chips, French fries, nuts, and nut butters) can exacerbate IC symptoms. High-oxalate foods can wreak havoc on some people's systems, and those with IC may be affected.

Oxalate is a compound that your body produces naturally, but it can also be found in a number of foods as it protects the crop from being eaten by insects. When oxalate in the body combines with calcium it can, under certain conditions, crystalize to form kidney or bladder stones. In certain people these crystals also irritate the body's sensitive tissue (such as bladder tissue) and cause or increase inflammation, leading to problems not just in the kidneys, but elsewhere. Ordinarily, oxalates will not cause the body too much trouble and are easily expelled from the body after digestion. However, in some people, especially those with gut issues or specific genetic variants, the oxalate is absorbed. This can lead to an oxalate over-absorption. Increased levels of oxalate can be found in the urine, blood, tissues, and even bone. In certain people, oxalates will not necessarily develop into actual kidney stones but can still irritate sensitive tissue, making a low-oxalate diet a preferable alternative.

Having excessive amounts of oxalate in the body can overwhelm your system, killing off *lactobacillus acidophilus* (helpful bacteria found mostly in the upper GI tract) and disrupting your gut flora, even if you are taking a daily probiotic. A number of IC sufferers have experienced relief from their symptoms after implementing a low-oxalate diet, along with many who suffer from kidney stones and gut problems.

This issue can be overcome by increasing your intake of calcium-rich, low-oxalate foods; drinking more water; and reducing your salt intake. Genetic testing will reveal whether or not variants are affecting the glyoxylate and hydroxypyruvate reductase (GRHPR) gene, which is responsible for converting oxalates. This can also be addressed with proper supplementation. Talk to your doctor for more information and a complete list of high-oxalate foods.

Nightshades

Finally, some people find nightshades (for example white potatoes, eggplant, tomatoes, chili peppers, and bell peppers) difficult to digest because they contain alkaloids, which may have an adverse effect on our health. They can cause inflammation as a result of excessive antibody production, thereby causing further digestive issues as well as headaches and joint pain. Avoiding nightshades will be necessary for some. Like everything else we have looked at, this will decrease the inflammatory response, which is always the goal.

These lists might seem overwhelming and discouraging, but take heart! Healing leaky gut can take months, but after that you may find you are no longer sensitive to the foods that once bothered you. Take things one day at a time and focus on making wise, healthy choices, starting from today.

Eat, eat, eat

We have been focusing on the foods you should not be eating, which can be frustrating, so let's regroup and give attention to what we should be eating. If we recognize that food is medicine, we will know that certain foods can decrease inflammation, heal the gut, reduce oxidative stress, and nourish the body. Fill your kitchen with the foods listed below and try to rotate them, because any kind of excess, for example eating eggs every day, may overwhelm your system and cause you to develop an intolerance.

Foods you should be eating:

- **Antioxidants (which reduce free radicals):** wild blueberries, dark chocolate, elderberries, artichokes, pecans, blackberries, sweet potatoes, kale, broccoli, strawberries, grapes, carrots, and cilantro.
- **Anti-inflammatory foods:** green leafy vegetables, almonds, beets, bok choy, broccoli, celery, walnuts, salmon, ahi, blueberries, strawberries, cherries, oranges, sprouted seeds, bone broth, coconut oil, and turmeric.
- **Fermented foods (good bacteria):** raw yogurt, kefir, kombucha, miso soup, sauerkraut, kimchi, pickles, and raw cheese.
- **Prebiotics (fiber):** raw dandelion greens, jicama, garlic, onions, leeks, Jerusalem artichokes, asparagus, and green bananas.
- **Cruciferous vegetables (which support detoxification, and decrease the risk of cancer):** arugula, Brussels sprouts, cabbage, collard greens, cauliflower, kale, radishes, broccoli, bok choy, and turnips.
- **Healthy fats:** avocado, coconut, organic dark chocolate (seventy percent cocoa), eggs, wild salmon, olive oil (unheated) and nuts (walnuts and almonds; soak beforehand, but refrain if on a low-oxalate diet).
- **Superfoods that should be bladder-friendly:** quinoa, blueberries, kale, chia, broccoli, strawberries, salmon, spinach, spirulina, eggs, almonds, ginger, beets, beans, pumpkin, apples, garlic, cauliflower, leeks, lentils, papaya, seaweed, black raspberries, parsley, arugula, avocado, Brussels sprouts, mango, turmeric, prunes, bok choy, and collard greens.

Why not follow a vegan or vegetarian diet?

The problem with following vegan and vegetarian diets is that most consume large quantities of grains including gluten, legumes, nuts, seeds, soy, and dairy (vegetarians only). Vegan and vegetarian diets may work for some people, but in others they can overwhelm the digestive system. Our bodies are capable of digesting unprocessed meats, and are able to absorb and use the nutrients found in animal meat, but the quality and quantity of meat we consume is crucial to our health. Organic, grass-fed meat, wild-caught fish, and free-range, organic poultry are full of nutrients, including protein, vitamins, minerals, and healthy fats.

Restoring balance to the body will open the door for you to be able to tolerate a wide variety of foods, which is important because we need the nutritional benefits found in many different food groups. Animal products offer high-quality protein compared with proteins found elsewhere, so avoiding them can lead to protein deficiency. This disrupts the liver's ability to detoxify, since it needs adequate nutrients in order to eliminate toxins from the body.

Finally, the fruit and vegetables we eat today are no longer as nutritious as they once were. Depleted soil, pesticides, fertilizers, and new varieties of crops have diminished the number of vitamins and minerals in our food. Having your own garden or purchasing organic fruits and vegetables from your local farmer's market is best, as is focusing on a balanced diet that consists of eating the right foods from a variety of food groups, in the correct portion sizes, and preparing them the right way. If you are a die-hard vegan or vegetarian, make sure you are eating foods that are high in amino acids. Since the body cannot produce the nine essential amino acids it needs, or store excess, you will need to make sure that your amino acid levels do not become depleted. Amino acids are crucial to your health and well-being as they play a role in digestion, hormone balance, and antibody management. They also serve to regulate the body's metabolic processes.

The biggest warning I will give here relates to soy. Soy is considered a complete protein because it contains the nine essential amino acids, but soy does not contain high levels of lysine and methionine. When you take into consideration the number of people struggling to digest it (intolerance) and the rise in allergies to it, soy really isn't a favorable substitute for high-quality animal protein. If you are consuming soy, make sure it is organic, because most soy is genetically modified and heavily saturated in pesticides, making it a terrible substitute for organic free-range poultry or grass-fed meat.

*

We have all heard the saying that knowledge is power, but I don't necessarily agree. It is definitely "potential power", but unless it's applied well – and coupled with action – knowledge is rendered useless. I wonder how long we will continue to turn a blind eye to the facts. How long will we ignore that which is right in front of us? When will we push off the laziness that so easily entangles us and decide to commit to a disciplined lifestyle? Of all the things we choose to compromise on, food cannot be one of them, and I'm talking to myself right now as much as to you! The diet we follow will affect our quality of life, as it plays an important role in our health, and in the illness that riddles our bodies. Let's take a peek at some of the foods and substances that are most likely to cause inflammation.

Wheat

Today, hybrid wheat makes up ninety-nine percent of the world's wheat, complete with new genetic strains. David Zivot, founder of GrainStorm, summed up the problem with our modern-day wheat perfectly when he said: "We have mutant seeds, grown in synthetic soil, bathed in chemicals. They're deconstructed, pulverized to fine dust, bleached and chemically treated to a create a barren industrial filler."

One of the most notable structural changes hybridization has on wheat is the genetic change of the gluten protein composite (the part that makes it doughy). Unfortunately, this change has brought with it a number of problems, including gluten intolerance and Celiac disease. I don't think manufacturers today care too much for the age-old adage "everything in moderation," because wheat is added to just about everything, to the extent that we are now being overexposed to it. Anything we consume in excess will bring negative consequences.

These new strains of wheat have been consumed by the vast majority of the population over the past fifty years, and the results are noteworthy. In his book, *Wheat Belly*, Dr. William Davis reports that modern-day wheat, which is a complex carbohydrate, increases blood sugar levels (more than a candy bar), which in turn increases blood insulin, causes irritability, and increases body weight (particularly visceral fat), since it converts to sugar. It can contribute to depression, gastrointestinal problems, fatigue, and increased appetite. It can trigger asthma and rashes, and disrupt pH balance. Furthermore, it can cause headaches, inflammation, and worsen ADHD and autism symptoms. If that were not enough, visceral fat or "belly fat," which is common in those who consume wheat, is linked to a host of other health conditions, including hypertension, diabetes, heart disease, dementia, colon cancer, rheumatoid arthritis, and abnormal insulin response. Bread, cake, cookie, and cracker cravings are fairly common for those who consume gluten because once it is broken down into gluten exorphins (peptides), opioid receptors in the brain are activated (drugs and sugar also do this), which causes us to crave more. This eventually results in addiction.

The reason I would recommend leaving wheat behind and opting for foods that are healthier is that the side-effects far outweigh the benefits. If gluten can cause inflammation or damage to the small intestine, why do we assume that it won't also affect the bladder? Indeed, gluten appears to be one of the worst offenders when it comes to inflammation. It lacks nutrients, disrupts hormones, and can cause or increase gut permeability. When the body doesn't recognize the gluten protein the immune system is triggered, which can elevate our antibody levels, triggering an autoimmune response.

If you are anywhere on the autoimmune spectrum, sensitive to gluten, or have digestive issues, including IBS, you should avoid gluten altogether, since it can wreak havoc on your gut as well as causing or contributing to chronic inflammation. The link between gluten and gut permeability is that when gluten is consumed it increases a chemical in the body called zonulin, which contributes to leaky gut because it causes the tight junctions in the intestinal walls to open up, allowing particles into the bloodstream. More than thirty percent of the U.S. population is sensitive to gluten (I personally believe this figure is much higher), and most people report an improvement after removing gluten from their diet. Humans lack the enzyme needed to digest modified grass, such as grains, and though many do not feel as though they have any trouble digesting gluten, this does not mean they are not being negatively affected by consuming it. Symptoms of gluten sensitivity include bloating, diarrhea, headaches, fatigue, inflammation, and skin rashes.

Rather than simply reducing our gluten intake, we should aim to eliminate it completely. Introducing even just a small amount back into the diet can scupper any progress made, as any consumption at all can spark an immune response, causing the inflammation to resurface. As gluten is the top inflammation-causing food, removing it from your diet is a given if you want to heal your gut and reduce inflammation in your bladder. It's important to understand that you are either gluten-free or you are not. There is no such thing as "mostly gluten-free." I know plenty of people who recognize that gluten is a trigger food for them, yet their mindset is that gluten isn't really that big of a deal as long as they eat less of it than they did before. Trigger foods are trigger foods, and an intolerance to gluten doesn't suddenly disappear just because you are eating reduced amounts.

After I removed gluten from my diet my bladder irritation decreased almost immediately, and oddly enough I actually have more energy without the sugar boost and subsequent crash. Initially, it will be difficult to leave the wheat behind, but if you take it one day at a time I promise it will get easier.

Some people find that they are able to tolerate sourdough or wheat from other countries, while others are sensitive and intolerant to all wheat. Sourdough manufacturers claim it is far more tolerable based on: a) evidence that the portion of lactobacillus to yeast in the sourdough leaven neutralizes the phytic acid in the wheat; b) that it takes longer to digest, which means it should not raise blood sugar levels as quickly or to such an extent compared with complex carbohydrates, which have a high glycemic index and are digested quickly, elevating blood sugar levels within minutes; and c) that it contains micronutrients due to the slow fermentation process, including zinc, iron, magnesium, and calcium, making these nutrients more available to the body and therefore a heathier option.

For those like my daughter, who find they are able to tolerate wheat grown in other countries, the problem may lie in the way wheat is grown and harvested here in the United States. This type of intolerance is likely due to a chemical intolerance rather than a gluten intolerance. Herbicides, fungicides, pesticides, and insecticides contain toxic ingredients, and detectable traces have been found in wheat flour, bread samples, rain, and urine. The biggest problem with modern-day wheat is its ability to disrupt good bacteria in the gut, disrupting the digestive system, promoting leaky gut, and overloading our immune systems. Even if you don't seem to react as badly to sourdough or imported wheat, the safest strategy is to cut it out altogether.

Dairy

Like most Americans, I assumed that cow's milk was created for human consumption, and I was part of the generation that grew up with the "Got milk?" commercials. This led me to believe that if I didn't drink milk regularly my bones would become so fragile they would eventually break off like Mr. Miller's. I was wrong! It's true that calcium is needed for healthy bones, but it turns out that milk, which is high in fat, is not the best source of calcium. We are better off forgoing dairy and instead eating calcium-rich foods such as beans, dark leafy greens, Brussels sprouts, lentils, figs, sesame seeds, and sardines. According to his book, *The Calcium Lie*, Dr. Robert Thompson, M.D., believes that focusing solely on calcium for strong bones can actually cause long-term consequences because dozens of minerals contribute to bone health, not just calcium. A delicate balance must be the goal in order for our bones to remain strong and healthy.

The problems with milk are numerous. First, due to overcrowded and unsanitary conditions, conventionally raised livestock are treated with antibiotics in order to prevent disease, contributing to the antibiotic resistance epidemic. Sanitary conditions are so grim that farming accounts for nearly eighty percent of antibiotic usage in the U.S. Little effort has been made to address this, leading to what has now become a major public health threat. According to the Federal Interagency Task Force: "The extensive use of antimicrobial drugs has resulted in drug resistance that threatens to reverse the medical advances of the last seventy years."

Second, dairy is a known allergen. Your body may "misread" it as a foreign invader, and on entering the bloodstream it will cause your immune system to create antibodies, triggering the release of histamine. This causes an inflammatory response, including inflammation of the bladder wall. Dr. Myers writes: "Unfortunately, your immune system's recognition system isn't perfect; as long as a molecule's structure is similar enough, your immune system registers it as an invader and attacks." Sometimes other proteins are "tagged" as gluten, and dairy products are the most commonly "misdiagnosed" because casein is very similar to the gliadin protein found in gluten. Dr. Myers claims that half of people with a gluten intolerance may also be sensitive to dairy for this reason. Other foods that may mistakenly trigger this response are corn, millet, oats, rice, and yeast.

"This process of cross-reactivity is also the same concept as the molecular mimicry phenomenon," Dr. Myers writes. "In both cases your immune system confuses innocent sources as invaders and begins to destroy them; however in the process of molecular mimicry, it's a part of your own body (such as thyroid tissue in those with Hashimoto's) that is being misidentified as an invader and attacked."

This means that simply giving up gluten, or giving up dairy, may not solve the problem, though these are good starting points. "Eating gluten (or gluten look-a-likes) can elevate your antibodies for up to three months, meaning that even if you only ate gluten or its cross-reactive foods four times a year, you would be in a state of inflammation year-round," she concludes.

Third, casein, a complex protein (which is chemically similar to gluten) found in dairy products, is difficult to break down and digest, which puts significant strain on the digestive system. Casein intolerance sometimes mimics the symptoms of those with a lactose intolerance.

Fourth, rennet, which causes milk to coagulate (and makes cheese hard), was once made from the lining of a calf's fourth stomach. However, due to supply and demand issues, most rennet is now genetically modified and should be avoided.

Fifth, dairy contains lactose and many people find they are lactose-intolerant because they do not make the enzyme lactase, which is needed to break down the lactose sugar found in cow's milk.

Added to this, consuming dairy produces acid, which will affect the pH balance in your body, as discussed earlier. In an attempt to compensate for this, alkalizing compounds including calcium, magnesium, and potassium are extracted from our bones, which can increase the risk of fractures and osteoporosis.

Dairy is the second-greatest inflammatory offender after gluten, and most people who are sensitive to gluten are also sensitive to dairy. This is due to reasons we already discussed and because gluten often damages the part of the intestine that produces lactase, an enzyme that breaks down lactose. Symptoms of dairy intolerance include abdominal cramps and bloating, acne, joint pain, IBS, diarrhea, and respiratory infections. Implementing a dairy-free diet has proven to help many IC sufferers by reducing bladder and intestinal inflammation. Some people who are sensitive to dairy are able to tolerate raw, grass-fed goat, camel, and sheep milk, and raw cheese or feta, while others may have to forgo all dairy and substitute with coconut, macadamia, cashew, or almond milk.

Refined sugar

Refined sugar, or "table sugar," comes either from sugar cane or genetically engineered (GE) sugar beets. During the refining process, sugar (sucrose, which contains glucose and fructose) is stripped of its minerals and nutrients, then bleached with either carbon dioxide or calcium hydroxide, leaving behind a white carbohydrate, which affects the way our bodies process and metabolize it. The end product consists not only of chemicals but of empty calories with no nutritional value.

Our bodies' cells, and particularly our brain cells, use glucose for energy, but fructose has a negative impact on the body. It neither stimulates insulin or leptin, nor inhibits ghrelin, which prevents us from feeling full and satisfied after eating. Fructose increases appetite and decreases metabolism, causing us to eat more and use up valuable mineral and vitamin stores to metabolize it. This makes us feel tired and lacking in energy, leading to cravings for more fructose. Sugar stimulates the brain, simulating dopamine production, which gives us a short-term buzz like certain narcotics, with the same addictive effects. Like the classic come-down after taking drugs, the blood sugar rush leads to a crash, which can make us feel lethargic as well as affecting mood, concentration, and digestion.

Perhaps most seriously, fructose has also been linked to insulin resistance, a forerunner of type II diabetes, which is sweeping the nation. It can increase uric acid levels, increasing our risk of gout, and raise blood pressure, which can lead to hypertension. It has also been linked to obesity, cancer, heart disease, liver disease, ADHD, tooth decay, and many other serious conditions. Finally, it can contribute to chronic inflammation, fueling autoimmune diseases and conditions such as IC.

Many of us consume vast quantities of sugar on a daily basis as it is added to so many products, ranging from ketchup to processed meats. The bladder can be negatively impacted even by moderate amounts of sugar. It disrupts gut flora by increasing the amount of yeast and bad bacteria in the small intestine, which produces toxins, causing or contributing to gut permeability and bladder irritation. Additionally, increased blood sugar levels will put you at a higher risk of developing a UTI, since any bacteria present in the urinary tract will feed off the sugar. Sugars and carbs (which act like sugar) change the ecosystem in your gut, feeding the growth of bad bacteria and setting you up for candida overgrowth.

It is best to forgo all refined sugars and artificial sweeteners if you can. Opt for unrefined sugar instead, which retains most of its minerals and nutrients, including calcium, iron, magnesium, potassium, and phosphorus. The best source is the natural sugar found in fruit and vegetables, but keep even this to a minimum, as it will increase your blood sugar levels and increase yeast and bacteria levels, albeit not as quickly as refined sugar. Raw honey, 100 percent pure maple syrup, Stevia, monk fruit, medjool dates, and coconut sugar are great alternatives, and are either completely natural or less refined than table sugar, making them a sweet substitute.

Grains and legumes

Healing your gut is a critical component in regaining your health. Therefore, you will need to remove anything and everything from your diet that puts extra stress on your digestive system, contributing to leaky gut. The chronic inflammation of IC is an immune response and, in order to relieve this current burden on your immune system, you may need to temporarily remove grains and legumes, which are difficult to digest.

We eat the part of the grain or legume that is actually the plant's seed, which was intended to be eaten by animals. After consumption it would be deposited further afield, still intact, giving the plant an opportunity to grow in fresh soil. Grains are comprised of complex proteins, but the issue here is that our bodies need to access the protein in its most basic form if we are to derive the nutrients we need from them. If not, we are unable to break it down and absorb it into our systems. While you may argue that our ancestors have been eating grains for countless years, the grains we eat today are almost entirely unrecognizable given the way they are grown and processed, which makes them significantly less nutritious than they might once have been. Added to this, many of us are massively over-consuming grains because they make our breads, cakes, pastries, crackers, and other processed foods moister and more delicious.

Tom and I recently returned from a trip to Europe, and we were surprised at how different the breads and pastries were over there. First of all, they were nowhere near as sweet, but we also found that in some countries they were dry and mealy (think corn bread, and not the one from Marie Callender's). One bite and it would crumble and fall apart. This was not the case in Paris – the pastry capital of the world – so I had to refrain from sweets and breads while we were there, but on the whole the European equivalents were easier to digest.

It may seem unrealistic or overwhelming to completely leave grains behind. It really is up to you, and whether or not your body is struggling to digest them. I recommend avoiding them while you detox and then reintroducing the right ones – in small quantities and prepared the correct way – to see if you are able to digest them with ease. Learning to prepare grains the way our ancestors did means that we sprout, ferment, or soak them prior to cooking. This helps to neutralize enzyme inhibitors. We need enzymes to break apart disaccharides (double sugars) and split them into single sugars, which can be digested and absorbed through the gut wall. Doing so also reduces "anti-nutrients." Grains are high in phytic acid, which inhibits digestion, resulting in decreased mineral absorption. Finally, preparing them the right way promotes the breakdown of complex proteins into simple proteins, which we are able to digest more easily, relieving the burden on the digestive tract.

Pesticides

Pesticides are often used on crops to kill or repel pests. Unfortunately, many are made with synthetic materials, and extreme exposure can lead to pesticide poisoning. Did you know that we have twenty-nine traceable pesticides inside our bodies right now, and the levels at which we are currently carrying them is unsafe? While the debate over their direct impact on humans rages on, studies have found that long-term exposure to pesticides, even in small quantities, is linked to a number of health conditions including cancer, infertility, and neurological defects. Chemicals used in the agricultural sector have neurotoxic properties that can alter our immune systems by decreasing the number of friendly microbes present, leading to food sensitivities and allergies.

The main ingredient of the most widely used herbicides is glyphosate, which is extremely controversial, and its usage has been completely banned in a number of countries. Multiple studies have been carried out since its introduction in 1974, but in the past few years studies have revealed a link between glyphosate and kidney disease, autism, cancer, Parkinson's, and Alzheimer's. Reports offered in defense by biotech companies do not contain accurate data. They minimize toxicity findings, since glyphosate testing is often undertaken in isolation from the other pesticides and chemicals used in the same mixture. However, when the toxicity of nine combined pesticides was undertaken, the results showed that eight were almost 1,000 times more toxic combined than when tested independently.

Bacillus thuringiensis (Bt) is a pesticide that was first used commercially in the U.S. in 1958, with only a dozen or so registered strains by 1977. There are thousands of strains of this spore-forming bacterium today, and these bacteria produce more than 200 protein crystals, which are toxic to a number of insects. In the late nineties, one pesticide manufacturer created a variety of corn that was resistant to its product, which contains glyphosate, by taking Bt-toxin from soil bacteria wash-off and putting the Bt-toxin gene into the seed. When an insect eats a plant containing Bt, the Bt-toxin produced inside the plant – which is far more poisonous than the spray – causes intestinal permeability by poking holes in the insect's intestine, allowing the toxin to enter its system and kill it.

The company was adamant that the toxin was not harmful to the digestive tract of humans or mammals, and assured the public that its new invention would only harm insects. However, studies have led scientists to believe that when humans consume GMOs, or livestock raised on GMOs, the Bt toxin has the potential to affect the integrity of the human digestive tract by poking holes in the intestine, causing intestinal permeability, or leaky gut. Researchers in Italy found that mice fed on Bt corn did, in fact, show alterations in their gut as well as an immune system response to the genetically modified corn, thereby indicating that GMOs cause inflammation in the body and should not be consumed by humans or livestock.

Organic produce is a far better option, although it may not be 100 percent organic unless labeled as such. Produce labeled "USDA organic" and "certified organic" must be at least ninety-five percent organic, with the remaining five percent meeting specific guidelines. Recent studies have found that organic crops possess higher volumes of antioxidants and flavonols, which decrease inflammation in the body while offering greater cell protection. Testing also showed that organic, grass-fed dairy and meat contained far more omega-3 fatty acids.

You can remove some pesticides by scrubbing your fruits and vegetables, then rinsing in a salt-water solution. Don't be tempted to wash meat, poultry, and eggs, however, as this can spread germs. Interestingly, pesticides are stored in animal fats, and cooking can actually increase pesticide levels in these proteins, further motivating consumers to purchase organic poultry and grass-fed beef.

GMO

Genetically modified organisms (GMOs) include plants, animals, and microorganisms that contain altered, man-made DNA rather than natural DNA obtained through mating or recombination. Americans were introduced to GMOs in 1996 and quickly began consuming them in significant quantities.

Insert or remove a single gene at a desired location and it alters an organism's DNA, allowing for a genetically engineered strain that is "tailored" to meet specific characteristics. Of course, we can be sure that whenever we decide to "improve" upon nature, everything always goes according to plan (eye roll). Unfortunately, when it came to genetic modification, scientists did not plan for a host of DNA gene mutations, or the side effects they would impose on humanity.

Though the invention of GMOs may have appeared wise, breeding strains of crops that make production easier, provide resistance to pesticides or viruses, withstand harsh weather conditions, have a longer shelf life, are more aesthetically desirable, or make herbicides tolerable could never be achieved without some risk to the human body. The vast majority of GMOs have been designed to tolerate herbicides, which has resulted in an increased use of herbicides. This has led to current problems with superweeds and superbugs that are resistant to the herbicides used, requiring stronger, more toxic poisons to get rid of them. According to a report by *The New York Times*, our GMO crops show that there is no discernible advantage in crop yields when measured against crops grown traditionally in parts of Europe. In the United States, GM crops include corn, cotton, soybeans, canola oil, sugar beets, papaya, zucchini, yellow squash, alfalfa, and Golden Delicious apples. Despite deafening shouts from the GMO companies in defense of their GM creations, it doesn't take a genius to see that something has gone awry.

We love cows here in America (though the commercial touting the fact that "Great cheese comes from happy cows. Happy cows come from California" is a lie), but a regular intake of milk, cheese, and meat should be avoided for a number of reasons. It is not uncommon for dairy cows to be injected with a GM growth hormone called rBST or rbGH, which serves to increase milk production. Nor is it unusual for cows, poultry, and swine to feed on genetically modified grains containing corn and soy. Always do your research and read your labels so you know what is in the food that you are consuming, and avoid products that contain GM ingredients, such as high fructose corn syrup (since it is derived from corn), soy-lecithin (an additive derived from soy that serves as an emulsifier), and certain GM yeasts found in wine. The FDA does not require companies to label GMOs, nor does it mandate that companies notify them prior to releasing them to the public. It is the consumers' responsibility to know what is in the food they are purchasing with regard to GMOs.

Unfortunately, genetic modification can have a hugely negative impact on the human body. If genetically modified food items produce new proteins they can potentially provoke an allergic reaction. While there is no firm evidence on this to date, studies are currently in progress and are likely to confirm that this is the case. Some of the genes contained in

GMOs may also increase our resistance to antibiotics, and if these genes are picked up by our gut bacteria further antibiotic resistance is likely to develop. Genetic modification may also increase toxin buildup in the body and affect digestion, making foods harder to digest and therefore less nutritious.

I believe that an anti-inflammatory diet must be coupled with a non-GMO diet if we are to experience rapid and lasting relief from our IC symptoms. According to the Institute for Responsible Technology (IRT), GMOs have been linked to a number of side effects, including "allergies, gluten intolerance, toxins, new diseases, nutritional problems, immune problems, accelerated aging, infertility, and changes in major organs and the gastrointestinal system." The IRT lists sixty-five health risks associated with GM foods, which you can find on its website (responsibletechnology. org). GMOs are potentially toxic, and are more than likely affecting our cells, organs, guts, immune systems, bodies, and lives. It's time to draw a line in the sand and refuse to tolerate anything less than organic, grass-fed meat and free-range poultry, as well as organic crops.

Is organic healthier?
Organic produce has been found to contain higher levels of antioxidants, including phenolic acids, flavones, and anthocyanins. These antioxidants are believed to reduce the risk of the very conditions pesticides are said to increase. Therefore, buying organic produce offers double benefits.

A study from RMIT University in Melbourne, Australia, showed an almost immediate ninety percent decrease in pesticide exposure when following an organic diet. The goal is always to reduce toxic exposure while increasing our intake of foods that are high in nutrients, so opt for fresh organic produce whenever possible.

How eating clean has worked for me
I decided to eliminate gluten, dairy, refined sugars, and GMOs from my diet, and to face the challenge of eating clean head on. At the end of the book you will find a five-day meal plan (see p. 141) to help you get off to a healthy start. Eating clean will require effort on your part, but it is definitely worth it. It can be life-changing in more ways than one.

The key here is to make every effort to eat as many vegetables as possible. Our plates should comprise two-thirds vegetables and one-third protein to provide us with the perfect balance. Vegetables are a great source of vitamins, minerals, and fiber, so increase your vegetable intake. The more colorful they are the better they will be for you. Try to eat your vegetables when they are fresh, and eat them raw so you get as many nutrients from them as possible. Summer fruit is still in season as I write, which makes following this diet fairly easy. When snacking, I reach for fresh fruits, veggies, nuts, or packaged organic snacks. Any snacks I bring into the house must be labeled organic at the top.

Being strategic with your diet will help to alleviate your IC symptoms as well as making you feel stronger and healthier overall. Begin reducing chronic bladder inflammation today by eliminating foods from your diet that have been deemed inflammatory, and seek to customize your diet so that is specific to your body's needs.

Chapter 8

METHYL GENETICS AND YOU

*"Our greatest weakness lies in giving up. The most certain way
to succeed is always to try just one more time."*

American inventor Thomas A. Edison

The future of medicine is personalized. In the not-too-distant future, treatments for all sorts of medical conditions will be tailored to your individual genetic profile: the unique DNA combination you inherited from your parents. The distinctive set of genetic instructions contained within each of your cells will also be targeted for preventative health measures, with customized methods developed to help prevent diseases that are identified as high-risk for your genetic makeup.

This process becomes slightly more complex when you factor in genetic variants. Every time a cell divides to form a new cell it sends the same genetic makeup with it. However, when variations occur and the new cell does not replicate in the exact same way, it produces a single nucleotide polymorphism (SNP).

SNPs are common, and everybody has them to some degree. The way each person's body reacts to its own SNPs will be unique. Most have little effect on a person's health or development. Still, by affecting the gene's function some SNPs play a significant role in disease, in circulatory and immune functioning, and in overall physical and emotional well-being. These genetic variants can have a significant impact when it comes to the main topic of this chapter: methylation.

What is methylation?
Methylation is a process that has already occurred billions of times within your body in the time it has taken you to read this. It is the process that essentially controls the replication of your DNA across every single cell

in your body. At its core, methylation occurs whenever the body adds a methyl group (consisting of one carbon and three hydrogen atoms) to a molecule. This ultimately changes how that molecule interacts with other substances in the body. Enzymes, genes, and hormones – all proteins subject to methylation – become altered through this process.

Without this intricate biochemical process, our well-being would be called into serious question. Take, for instance, the toxic amino acid homocysteine. Methylation can transform homocysteine into methionine, an amino acid that is beneficial to our bodies. Without methylation, toxins continue to build up in our bloodstream, which sets off the process of inflammation and chronic illness.

As with most other interdependent biochemical processes in our bodies, methylation is necessary for subsequent reactions to take place, including RNA and DNA synthesis, the regeneration of creatinine, and immune responses that protect us from illnesses.

Methylation plays a role in everything from our behavior and mood regulation to concentration, memory, and sleep, all through the synthesis of neurotransmitters. Methylation helps support our health and development through the myelination and pruning of nerves. Myelination contributes to the growth of a protective covering of our body's nerve fibers, while pruning facilitates more complex mental function by shedding older synapses and making space for higher-quality new ones. Without proper methylation levels, our bodies cannot perform either process effectively, which means that our nervous systems will not be able to function properly.

Methylation also affects the performance of our enzymes and genes. All the chemical reactions that are required in order for us to digest food, along with the metabolic processes in our cells and tissues, require enzymes. Methylation contributes to gene expression, meaning it can essentially lock our genes into the "on" or "off" position through epigenetic signaling. Depending on the specific gene, this could either be beneficial or detrimental to our health.

A DNA test can help to reveal your genetic predispositions to certain diseases, such as cancer or mental illness. Turning off genes so they are not expressed could actually help to reduce your risk of developing those diseases. However, where there is poor methylation there is an increased risk when it comes to a range of different health conditions and chronic illnesses, including:

- ADD/ADHD
- Allergies
- Alzheimer's disease
- Autism
- Cancer
- Chronic fatigue syndrome
- Chronic migraines
- Difficulty fighting off infections
- Digestive issues
- Fibromyalgia
- Frequent miscarriages
- Heart attacks
- IBS
- Infertility
- Mood disorders
- Multiple sclerosis
- Neuropsychiatric disorders
- Parkinson's disease
- Spina bifida
- Stroke

In short, methylation keeps us healthy. It can help keep our immune systems strong, repair our cells and tissues, control gene expression, regulate our hormones, detoxify our bodies, and keep our energy levels high. However, genetic mutations often disrupt the methylation process, making it harder for the body to do its job.

The good news is that, thanks to evolving research, we now know that genetic factors account for fewer than ten percent of all illnesses. This means the environmental factors we are exposed to from the time we are born, and the way these factors interact with our genes, account for the remaining ninety percent. Why is that good news? Because it means we have more control over our health than we once realized.

Despite an inherited predisposition to certain conditions our health is primarily in our own hands. Through a healthy diet, limiting our exposure to environmental toxins, and taking the correct nutritional supplements, we can help suppress the expression of those genetic mutations and launch a strong counterattack on illnesses before they strike. The road to good health is in front of us.

DNA

According to DNA research, the root cause of most illnesses can be traced back to two factors: the presence of free radicals, including superoxide and peroxynitrite; and oxidative stress. Glutamate and ammonia can also damage our systems. However, our bodies naturally produce all these elements. The problem lies in poor methylation due to genetic variants, which can lead to an overgrowth of free radicals. This ultimately leads to inflammation and cell damage, which not only makes it harder for your body to repair its cells but can actually speed up the aging process and make your body ripe for disease.

That is why the body keeps busy producing antioxidants, including superoxide dismutase, catalase, and glutathione, to help repair and rebuild those damaged cells. However, our genetic variants may be holding us back. On top of causing us to produce too many oxidants they may also be hampering our ability to create antioxidants or the folate we need to repair cells. Additionally, variants can affect our ability to break down histamine and may impact the production of cellular energy.

If you take a DNA test your saliva will produce some amazing insights relating to 602,000 pieces of DNA. The results will reveal your capacity to make and use the enzymes you need for total health, including:

- B12: to make blood cells and support a healthy nervous system
- BH4: to support neurotransmitters and detoxify ammonia
- Choline: to improve liver function
- Glutathione: to eliminate toxins and control inflammation
- SAMe: to support a range of healthy bodily functions
- SOD: to neutralize the superoxide radical
- Folate: to improve neurotransmitter and cellular health
- Neurotransmitters: to support emotional health

MTHFR

MTHFR is a gene that produces methyl folate, and subsequently tells your body how to break down the homocysteine amino acid (which we have already established is toxic). The MTHFR mutation, or SNP, is typically associated with poor methylation. However, as knowledge surrounding MTHFR continues to evolve we must consider it alongside all the other genes that contribute to the methylation process as we seek to understand the role they each play.

Detox and immune function

Methylation is especially critical in today's world for its detoxifying properties and impact on our immune systems. As we become more exposed than ever before to environmental toxins we need to seek out ways to restore inner balance and purity, and to restore this equilibrium. Methylation is one of the major pathways through which detoxification occurs in our bodies. Without proper methylation the process of detoxification can be impaired. Toxins, including heavy metals, can build up in the body and contribute to a host of other health risks. This can also make it more difficult to recover from conditions such as SIBO and chronic yeast overgrowth. There is research linking poor methylation levels to autoimmunity, but more work is needed in this area.

Testing

If you are interested in learning more about your genetic makeup, or want to find answers to any of the health challenges you face, why not consider having your DNA tested? Doing so will allow you to identify your unique SNPs and the related nutritional weaknesses that are occurring in your body.

A simple genetic saliva test (try Your Genomic Resource from tolhealth. com) will set you on the path toward a customized treatment plan. Trained professionals will be able to analyze your data whichever kit you use, including the discontinued 23andMe test (visit gettoknowyourDNA. com to find a service in your area).

Once you have the results your health adviser can help identify your nutritional deficiencies and provide you with a nutritional protocol tailored to your unique needs. This protocol will supplement any missing nutrients and antioxidants, or will use nutrients and herbs to produce the enzymes you need to support healthy cells and reduce damaging oxidants.

The report is broken down into nine categories:

1. Gut health
2. Cellular energy production
3. Antioxidant and detoxification
4. Folate
5. Methionine cycle
6. Transsulfuration pathway
7. Neurotransmitters

8. BH4, urea cycle, nitric oxide (genetic variants may impact the clearing of toxins and the production of helpful molecules)
9. Miscellaneous items

Dr. Deckert says: "After much research I made the decision to purchase a program called Genetics Made Simple, which looks at hundreds of SNPs and groups them according to which pathway or systems in the body they might affect. The man behind the research is Dr. Robert Miller, a certified naturopath (CTN). To my knowledge, no one else out there is taking genetic influences on health to this level. He developed, and is still developing, Functional Genomic Nutrition Analysis software, which gives practitioners access to educational materials and enables us to analyze our genetic makeup.

"Beneath the ancestry and medical information given, the raw data of thousands of genes is recorded. This data is then uploaded into the MethylGenetic software, which allows the practitioner to look at multiple reports relating to any SNPs identified. It also provides a questionnaire for the patient to fill out so their symptoms can be correlated with the pathways that may be affected by multiple SNPs. Taking all this information into consideration, I explain to my patients the pathways that look as though they may be affected based on the laboratory data and the symptoms survey. I have found this information invaluable for my own health and the health of my patients.

"Dr. Miller has also designed a line of products that nutritionally support the pathways that may be affected. These products are formulated by Professional Health Products, which is well known for its glandular and homeopathic remedies. When a patient's report is complete, the pyramid he or she has formulated shows the clinician where to start, which often involves diet and lifestyle changes. Many of the body's pathways affect inflammation, and it is vital for me to help patients quench the fire burning within them. This research helps us understand why they are on fire and how to combat the flames. Doing so relates to all the other chapters discussed in this book, and will play a significant role in overcoming chronic illness. To find a trained health care professional near you who understands how to support genetic variants with nutrition go to gettoknowyourdna.com."

The information I have laid out in this book is what I believe to be the key to not only addressing IC but also chronic inflammation and autoimmune disease in general. For me, addressing genetic variants by providing a nutritional workaround played a significant role in sending my interstitial cystitis into remission. Methylation is a very important piece of the puzzle and is one of the factors behind IC, fibromyalgia, gut permeability, neurological issues, chronic fatigue, chronic infections, nervous system malfunctions, cognitive function, and an overburdened detoxification system. There are effective ways to deal with these issues, so speak with a trained health care professional who can help you with methyl genetic nutrition and complete the missing piece of the IC puzzle.

As I mentioned earlier, I tested positive for the MTHFR gene mutation A1298C a few years ago. After an initial flare-up the 5-MTHF (folate) and Methyl-B12 shots served to reduce the chronic inflammation, strengthen my immune system, decrease adrenal fatigue, and minimize my IC symptoms. I was shocked to say the least!

From there, Dr. Deckert ran further genetic testing and provided me with genetic nutrition to help pathways that were struggling. I found tremendous success with the shots, but we now understand that this is not the best place to start. If you have gone though the steps laid out above – including detox, gut repair, and diet changes – and still feel you are struggling with IC symptoms I would certainly recommend genetic testing.

Chapter 9

STRESS, HORMONES, AND BACTERIAL INFECTIONS

*"Strength does not come from physical capacity.
It comes from an indomitable will."*

Indian philosopher Mahatma Gandhi

"Stress can kill you" is a phrase my husband loves to share with me whenever he sees me stressed out over something or other. Our stress levels, the way we cope with stress, and more importantly how we think about stress, have a direct effect on our health, mental well-being, and spirit. I'm sure that you have made the connection between stress and increased bladder symptoms, or more specifically with flare-ups. Whenever I went on vacation my IC symptoms fell to an all-time low compared with the rest of the year. Away from the daily stress and pressures of life my mind and body relaxed, and my bladder calmed itself down. This affirmed to me that stress was a cofactor in the condition that had ravaged my body for more than a decade.

There is reason to believe that a person with IC may possibly have a nervous system that is in a state of "hyper stress," which contributes to IC and its symptoms. Cortisol is known as "the stress hormone," and our cortisol levels spike when we are in a stressful or dangerous situation. This produces a "fight or flight" response, which was designed to protect us from danger by alerting us to respond to a situation immediately. Once we are no longer in that situation our cortisol levels should return to normal. Unfortunately, many of us today are leading stressful lives and carrying burdens we were not meant to carry alone. Perhaps you have experienced a traumatic event that has left you with post-traumatic stress disorder (PTSD), or maybe you have experienced a prolonged period in which you had to endure constant stress due to a specific situation or chronic pain.

This may have resulted in a continuously heightened state of stress, which the body identifies as a threat.

When we become stressed out our adrenal glands produce adrenaline, norepinephrine, and cortisol. When we are constantly stressed, our raised cortisol levels may become chronic, negatively affecting the body by suppressing the immune system, disrupting thyroid function, increasing our appetite, impairing the body's ability to absorb crucial vitamins and minerals from food, and disrupting our sleep. On the other hand, if our cortisol levels are too low the adrenal glands become fatigued. This can lead to dizziness, fatigue, decreased appetite, and palpitations.

There's a direct connection here, because adrenal function correlates with gut and liver function. Leaky gut causes toxins to overburden the liver, which reduces the body's ability to handle the chemicals we use on a daily basis. Inflammation in the small intestines causes the adrenal glands to produce huge quantities of cortisol in an attempt to suppress inflammation. So, over time, gut permeability diminishes adrenal function. There will initially be an adrenal excess, but in the long run cortisol levels will drop and exhaustion will inevitably follow. The body then starts "borrowing" from progesterone stores to maintain the cortisol levels needed to handle the inflammation caused by leaky gut. This can lead to estrogen dominance because our progesterone levels have dipped too low to maintain the balance.

Cortisol is primarily responsible for how well the body copes with stress, and an inability to regulate cortisol levels can result in a number of health issues. Additionally, leaky gut will affect serotonin levels, and genetic variants will affect certain pathways and their ability to regulate stress.

Chronic stress must be addressed, since leaving it unchecked can lead to abnormal adrenal function, exacerbating IC symptoms in a body that is already in a fragile state. Furthermore, stress can cause the muscles in our bodies to tense up, specifically in the tightening of the pelvic floor muscles. This can further irritate the bladder.

Cortisol should be tested by saliva and collected four times in one day for the most accurate results. Blood tests can determine whether or not your adrenal function is within normal range, so talk with your doctor about testing cortisol levels, hormone levels, thyroid function, and neurotransmitters. I have added neurotransmitter testing because neurotransmitters play an important role in terms of the way chemical messengers transmit messages between our cells, and this process is also affected by chronic stress. The genetic testing I underwent revealed that certain genetic variants were affecting the production and breakdown of neurotransmitters, which control my mood; specifically the genes that control serotonin, dopamine, and glutamate, which can result in anxiety if this is not addressed.

In light of this, I began taking supplements to offer these enzymes support, and within a week my entire body felt much calmer. I recently added in Cortisol Manager for about a month. This is a stress hormone stabilizer from Integrative Therapeutics, which promotes healthy cortisol levels. Coupling these supplements with stress management therapy has literally enabled me to breathe deeply again. The way we manage stress in our lives is critical; not just to the state of our bladders, but to our overall heath.

For most of my life I have been unable to handle stress well, as I became anxious whenever I found myself in a stressful situation. This would send my bladder into a flare-up within five to ten minutes, and bringing my stress levels down required conscious effort on my part. For the most part I have learned to manage my stress by talking it through with someone I love, going for a walk and getting some fresh air, practicing my yoga breathing techniques, prayer, yoga, or going to the gym. Any of these options work for me, and all of them require me to momentarily step back from the situation. With this set intention, stress no longer has the hold on me that it once had, and I am better for it. Supplementation without the implementation of regular exercise will not be enough to bring about quick and lasting change, but a combination of the two, along with a healthy diet, might just transform your life.

The last supplement I added to my routine was OptiMag Neuro, described as "patented Magnesium for the brain." Magnesium helps with anxiety and panic attacks by keeping adrenal stress under control. It also serves as a natural blood thinner. Magnesium deficiency is a contributing factor in asthma, blood clots, bowel disease, cystitis (bladder spasms), depression (serotonin levels), diabetes, fatigue, heart disease, hypertension, hypoglycemia, insomnia, kidney disease, migraines, musculoskeletal conditions (such as fibromyalgia), nerve problems, PMS, osteoporosis, Raynaud's syndrome, and tooth decay. Magnesium L-Threonate is the only form of magnesium that has been proven in animal studies to cross the blood-brain barrier. It boosts the brain's magnesium levels, making it vital to healthy cognition. This encompasses long and short-term memory, learning, stress management, and sleep.

It has helped tremendously with my mood (anxiety and stress), and I now feel calmer than I have in my entire life, plus I'm sleeping like a baby. It's strange that you can go your whole life struggling with something like stress and anxiety, and try as you may to bring it under control the inward battle rages on. Well, that is no longer the case! Magnesium has had a tremendous effect on my life, my IC, my stress levels, my serotonin levels, and my cognition. You wouldn't think a deficiency here would have had such a broad effect on my overall wellness, but it did. Thank you, Dr. Deckert, for placing it in my hands. I am more than grateful! Right now, this is my absolute favorite supplement.

Hormones
Hormones are chemical messengers that move through the body and coordinate a range of complex processes. As they are involved in almost every function of the body, a hormone imbalance can make you feel bloated, tired, stressed, and depressed. Below are ten common symptoms that may indicate a hormone imbalance.

Irregular periods and bad PMS
It's normal for our hormone levels to shift before and during a period or pregnancy, or while going through perimenopause (the period before menopause), or menopause. But if you have irregular periods, you may be suffering from a hormone imbalance. The same applies if your PMS symptoms, or the pain and bleeding you experience at the time of your period, are severe. Alternatively, you could be suffering from a condition such as polycystic ovarian syndrome (PCOS), so it's important that you get to the bottom of the problem.

Sleep issues
Trouble getting to, or staying, asleep can be another indication of hormone imbalance. If your progesterone (a hormone released by your ovaries) levels are lower than they should be, this may make it more difficult to get a good night's sleep. Meanwhile, low estrogen levels can cause hot flashes and night sweats, which can make healthy sleep more elusive. If you're sleeping well but feel constantly fatigued, your progesterone levels may be too high or you may not be producing enough thyroid hormone.

Attention and memory problems
Hormone imbalance may also cause your brain to feel "foggy". Changes to your estrogen and progesterone levels can affect your alertness and memory. Some experts believe estrogen may affect the brain's neurotransmitters, which explains why memory and attention levels can be impacted during perimenopause and menopause. While other hormone-related conditions such as thyroid disease or adrenal issues could be the main cause, it's worth investigating if you are struggling to think clearly.

Digestive issues
There are many factors that could contribute to digestive issues, but as the gut is lined with tiny cells called "receptors" that respond to estrogen and progesterone, changes to our hormone levels can affect digestion. Perhaps you're suffering from bloating, stomach pain, nausea or diarrhea before or during your period. If there is a link with your hormone levels, your doctor may recommend some form of hormone therapy.

Changes to your breasts
Low estrogen levels can make your breast tissue less dense, while high levels can thicken this tissue, which may even cause lumps or cysts. If you notice changes to your breasts or experience severe pain, particularly just before or during your period, get this checked out. It's not normal for your breasts to feel tender every month before your period, and this may be a sign that you're having problems with estrogen metabolism.

Headaches
While there are many causes of headaches, some women experience headaches before or during their period, when estrogen levels are dropping.

Chronic acne
While breakouts are fairly common during a period, severe or chronic acne may be a symptom of hormone imbalance. High levels of androcens ("male" hormones that everyone has) can cause our oil glands to work overtime. These hormones can also affect the skin cells in and around our hair follicles, causing painful acne and clogged pores.

Depression and mood swings
Changes to your hormone levels may cause low mood, mood swings, and

even depression. Estrogen has an impact on your brain's chemicals, such as dopamine, serotonin, and norepinephrine. Other hormones can also affect the way we feel, so it's worth investigating your hormone levels if you're feeling low.

Sex-related problems

Loss of libido and vaginal dryness have been linked to hormone imbalance. If your testosterone levels are low, you may find that you have a lower sex drive than usual. If your estrogen levels are low, your body may produce less vaginal fluid. This can cause inflammation and tightness, making sex uncomfortable or even painful. It could also lead to urinary leakage.

Appetite changes and weight gain

If your estrogen levels dip, you may feel like eating more than you usually would. Many women feel the need to comfort eat, as an estrogen dip can affect our leptin levels, which regulate food intake and appetite. This can lead to unexpected weight gain and obesity.

When trying to connect the dots, hormonal balance and transitions must factor in our overall strategy for well-being. Hormones do not act alone, so treating them in isolation from the rest of the body is never a sensible approach. This is because hormones are not linear. They work in a number of bodily functions, since hormone imbalance is a key contributing factor to your IC symptoms.

It's worth speaking to your doctor if you are experiencing any of the symptoms listed above. It might be that your condition is not related to your hormone levels, but it's vital that you get to the root cause either way. Some medications and medical conditions can also cause your hormone levels to rise or fall, so find a doctor who will look at the bigger picture, and who will use biodentical hormones to help restore balance when needed.

Bacterial infections

Remember when I shared my first attempt at curing myself of IC by taking a large dose of antibiotics? At the time, a urine broth culture was not an available option in determining whether or not I had streptococcus. I forged ahead without the test and took two rounds of the antibiotic Doxycycline, to no avail. Though an occult (hidden) bacterial infection was not contributing to my IC symptoms, there is evidence that the infectious organisms staphylococcus aureus and streptococcus D (a form of enterococcus) are present in a significant percentage of those with IC.

Ordinarily, a healthy immune system and a healthy bladder mucosa provide resistance against these infectious agents, with antibodies presenting a strong line of defense. Unfortunately, when one of these organisms comes up against a weakened immune system, a leaky gut, and a damaged bladder, supported by a poor diet, the bacteria can breed and thrive, creating a bacterial infection, which is often painful. I believe these infectious organisms contribute to IC symptoms; however, if you have tried everything laid out in this book and are still not getting to the root of your IC, consider asking your doctor to order a urine broth culture to determine whether or not these organisms are present.

I would advise you to proceed with great caution if your results are positive, because treating them with antibiotics is inadvisable due to the fact that they can really damage your gut. They can wreak havoc on your immune system, disrupt gut flora, and lead to antibiotic resistance. To counter some of these issues you will require probiotics, IgG support, antifungals (coconut oil can be used topically as an antifungal), vitamins, supplements, and a large dose of patience. My advice is to treat antibiotics as a last resort when all else has failed because the side effects can be serious and should be carefully considered.

Antimicrobial alternatives
Before you decide to give antibiotics a go, there are other options. Much of the world depends on herbal remedies for healthcare remedies.

Black seed oil
Black seed (nigella sativa) is a flowering plant native to South Asia, and it is used to treat a broad spectrum of health issues. This ancient remedy demonstrates antimicrobial activity, including an inhibitory effect on staphylococcus aureus. Rumored to "cure everything but death" (though this is quite a stretch), black seed oil has been proven to be effective against ten strains of pathogenic bacteria and yeast, as well as possessing medicinal properties. It is said to be anti-rheumatic, anti-inflammatory, and anti-asthmatic. It supports the immune system, aids digestion, and relieves

hypertension and dermatological conditions, as well as helping in cancer prevention and treatment, and in the treatment of diabetes.

I purchased organic, cold-pressed black seed oil on Amazon. I mix two teaspoons with a glass of water and drink it every day, but you can also put it on your salad. The person who made me aware of black seed oil said that she pours it over her avocado every morning. Either way, the benefits to your overall health make it worth the momentarily unpleasant taste, which you must learn to get past in order to reap its rewards. Further information about black seed oil can be found on Dr. Axe's website (draxe.com).

Oil of oregano

Oil of oregano (*Labiatae*) is nature's own antibiotic and provides a proven healing compound. This powerful and well-known remedy consists of thymol and carvacrol, which have antibacterial and antifungal properties. It is also known to aid gastrointestinal health, reduce inflammation, combat candida, and deal with parasites. Because I was working to heal leaky gut, I incorporated a round of oil of oregano for fourteen days to treat any parasites or bacteria that might have taken up residence due to a compromised immune system, gut permeability, and a damaged bladder lining.

Grapefruit seed extract

Next time you eat a grapefruit make sure you don't throw away the seeds. Those seeds, especially in the form of grapefruit seed extract (GSE), offer a powerhouse of health benefits. If you don't have access to seeds the supplement is also available online through major sellers such as Amazon. GSE can help not only in UTI treatment but in everything from earaches and throat infections to candida and diarrhea. GSE contains elements that are antibacterial, antifungal, and antiviral all at once.

With candida, for instance, GSE helps kill the yeast cells that have overgrown in your body. Similarly, with fungal infections such as histoplasmosis, GSE can help fight infection by making the immune system stronger. It has also been known to treat imbalances in your gut bacteria, and can even be used as a general antimicrobial.

Other natural remedies

Corn silk tea is recognized as one of the most natural remedies for urinary problems and may be effective in reducing IC symptoms. It is believed to flush out toxins, reducing inflammation in the bladder, kidneys, and liver. Sweet and easy to make, it can have a noticeable effect without even tasting like medicine! Marshmallow root tea is also excellent in helping to soothe interstitial tissue and IC discomfort. It helps to coat the damaged bladder lining, reducing redness and swelling, as well as killing bacteria, speeding up the healing process, and helping to repair the lining of the gut.

Turmeric is another of nature's gifts that contains a wide variety of health benefits. I have incorporated the supplement into my daily regimen and started cooking with it whenever possible. This medicinal herb is one of the world's most powerful, as it contains anti-inflammatory healing properties while also being rich in antioxidants that are proven to help in reducing pain, as well as with diabetes management, skin conditions, gastrointestinal issues including IBS, controlling inflammation, and relieving oxidative stress. It can also help to treat cancer.

Talk with your doctor about incorporating one or more of these natural remedies into your healthcare routine. This may require long-term use as well as a cycling through these remedies in order to fully address your issue with pathogens. You may even want to consider a combination of natural remedies before falling back on antibiotics.

Chapter 10

THE ONGOING JOURNEY TO BETTER HEALTH

"Take the first step in faith. You don't have to see the whole staircase, just take the first step."

Baptist minister and activist Martin Luther King, Jr.

Seeking to take care of your whole body is one of the greatest gifts you can give yourself. We simply aren't our best selves when we are warring against health issues, which can easily consume us. Sometimes we need to be reminded that these issues do not only affect us; they also touch the lives of others. This should give us the energy and determination we need to make changes in our lives for our own betterment and the betterment of our families.

To a certain extent you are in control of how you live your life, what you consume, and how you spend your time. If you are serious about getting healthy and reclaiming your life, you will do just that. No excuse will cause you to detour from your goals. After you have detoxed, healed your gut, implemented a clean diet that is specific to your body's unique requirements, and added the proper supplementations based on your genetic testing, your journey to better health will require you to pursue the next step to wellness for the rest of your life.

Right now, conventional medicine treats women the same way it has for the last two decades when it comes to the health of their breasts. We need to seriously re-evaluate the use of mammograms as the number-one tool in detecting breast cancer. The fact that a more effective alternative for early detection exists but is rarely recommended is somewhat mind-boggling. Let me just state that I am not opposed to modern medicine, and it certainly has its place within society. In many cases it is life-saving, in fact. Modern medicine has made a huge contribution to advances in human health, enabling us to treat disease, illness, and injury much more effectively. My issue lies in the fact that, more often than not, conventional medicine offers symptomatic management instead of addressing the underlying causes of many health issues. I strongly believe that addressing the root cause of an issue and actively pursuing preventative care for patients is where true health and healing take place.

Thermographic testing

Thermographic testing uses digital infrared imaging to produce high-resolution images of temperature variations in the body. This allows metabolic changes and increased blood vessel activity to be detected, as it is able to measure minute temperature changes. These "biomarkers" can be used to assess health and detect body imbalances some six to eight years earlier than any other medical tests.

Unlike mammograms, thermal imaging is noninvasive, does not involve radiation, and is 100 percent safe. This diagnostic system makes it possible to detect a number of conditions including (but not limited to) inflammation, lymphatic congestion, body toxicity, kidney conditions, cardiovascular health, and autoimmune disorders. Early detection is crucial, and thermography detects inflammation, which is a precursor to most degenerative diseases. Therefore, it provides patients with the opportunity to begin preventative care long before symptoms have manifested.

I had the pleasure of being referred to Catherine Johnson, C.C.T., who conducted a thermal imaging scan on me at Silk Thermal Imaging in San Diego. The appointment was relatively quick, but our conversation around the importance of early detection, the benefits of thermography, and maintaining a healthy diet lingered. Upon listening to the benefits of thermography I became burdened not only for those around me but also for the many women relying on mammograms alone to inform them about the status of their health. If detection is possible in the early stages, or even long before cancer has developed, why are doctors choosing not to protect their patients' health?

I don't want to wait for symptoms to bear testament to the fact that something is amiss. I want a clear picture, and I want as much foreknowledge as is humanly possible! I understand that having 100 percent control over my health is not possible, as I do not hold my life in my own hands, but I want to do my best to take care of my body. After all, I only get one shot at this life, and I want to make the most of the gift I have been given. I want to be informed about what is going on and the options available outside of that which has been deemed "traditional" or "conventional." I have committed to having a thermal scan once a year going forward. Please consider taking this next step with me and find a reputable thermal imaging facility near you.

External influences

Since our goal is to reduce environmental toxins and alleviate the toxic burden on our immune systems, it is important to discuss some of the products we use on a daily basis, from cleaning products to makeup. Many of these contain ingredients that are harmful to our bodies. Resist the inclination to close your eyes and ignore what is going on around you, or in this case *inside* you. Educate yourself, do some research, and find out which ingredients your shampoo, cosmetics, and perfumes contain.

Beauty products are not regulated by the Food and Drug Administration (FDA), which has resulted in 1,300 chemicals that are banned in the E.U. being permitted in U.S. products. Testing has shown that many of these toxic ingredients, which are absorbed into the bloodstream upon usage, contain carcinogens. They can cause hormone disruption and neurotoxicity, resulting in cancer, lung damage, and other harmful effects on the body. I do not want to go into great detail here, so I will let you research it for yourself; however, parabens should be avoided at all costs.

According to *Prevention Magazine*'s *Eat Clean, Stay Lean*, parabens, which can be found in our cosmetics "mimic estrogen and could increase your risk of breast cancer." Other ingredients that should be avoided include: phthalates (a group of chemicals used to make plastic more flexible), dibutyl phthalate (DBP, a plasticizer), toluene (an aromatic hydrocarbon), petroleum-based chemicals, beta hydroxy acid (BHA), diethanolamine (DEA), sodium lauryl sulfate (SLS), and dioxane (a heterocyclic organic compound). This is not a full list, but all these chemicals can cause problems, and we need to demand that cosmetic, skincare, and cleaning product companies begin using healthy ingredients in the products we use.

As women, we tend to take our beauty regimens pretty seriously in an attempt to slow down the aging process by just about any means possible, but we may not realize that the beauty products we pay an arm and a leg for contain an average of 168 chemicals (including lead). We absorb traces of these every time we spray, pat, smear, rub, or dab them onto our skin. Read your labels, do your research and find out what is in your products!

Healthier alternatives

Below are some of the products I have found to offer high quality levels with little or no chemical component. If you want to continue to use cosmetics and cleaning products, try to opt for the following or similar alternatives:

Acne treatment: Countercontrol SOS Acne Spot Treatment by Beautycounter (beautycounter.com)

Air purifiers: GermGuardian high-efficiency particulate air and charcoal air purifiers (guardiantechnologies.com)

Bed linens: Organic bedding from No Feathers Please (nofeathersplease.com)

Body soap: citrus soap from Green Bath & Body (begreenbathandbody.com), or herbal body wash from Elina Organics (elinaorganicsskincare.com)

Cleaning products: buy from GreenShield Organic (greenshieldorganic.com), Planet All Purpose (planetinc.com), or Seventh Generation (seventhgeneration.com)

Cookware: buy from GreenPan (greenpan.com), Scanpan (scanpan.com), or Instant Pot (instantpot.com)

Deodorant: buy from Primal Pit Paste (primalpitpaste.com)

Laundry detergent and fabric softener: buy from Eco-Me (eco-me.com), GreenShield (greenshieldorganic.com), or Planet Ultra (planetinc.com)

Dishwasher liquid: buy from Planet Ultra (planetinc.com)

Face Moisturizer: Hyaluronic Serum from Be Natural Organics (benaturalorganics.com), or any of Elina Organics' moisturizers (elinaorganicsskincare.com)

Face wash: Mineral Face Wash from Luxe Heavenly Bodies (lhb-usa.com), or any of Elina Organics' face washes (elinaorganicsskincare.com)

Feminine hygiene products: organic, non-GMO cotton, chlorine-free, fragrance-free, deodorant-free from Seventh Generation (seventhgeneration.com), LOLA (mylola.com), or Cora (cora.life)

Lip balm: Primal Pucker Paste from Primal Pit Paste (primalpitpaste.com)

Makeup: buy from 100% Pure (100percentpure.com),

W3ll People (w3llpeople.com), or La Bella Figura (labellafigurabeauty.com)

Body moisturizer: Organic Shea Butter from Be Green Bath & Body (begreenbathandbody.com)

Nail polish: buy from butter LONDON (butterlondon.com), 100% Pure (100percentpure.com), or ella+mila's Elite Collection (ellamila.com)

Shampoo: NaturOli's Extreme Soap Nut/Soap Berry shampoo (naturoli.com), argan oil shampoo, or Herbal Healing shampoo from Elina Organics (elinaorganicsskincare.com)

Sunscreen: Juice Beauty's SPF 30 Sport Moisturizer (juicebeauty.com), or Pacific Beach Organics' Broad Spectrum (pacificbeachorganics.com)

Toothpaste: Revitin's prebiotic toothpaste (revitin.com)

Water filtration system: Radiant Life's 14-Stage Biocompatible Water Purification System (radiantlifecatalog.com)

Wrinkles: avoid Botox and fillers; instead, try Rezenerate, which stimulates the production of collagen and elastin; or a microcurrent facial, which uses an electrical current to help lift, firm, and tone sagging facial muscles.

Plastics and cookware

By now, we are all aware that we should be using plastics that are free of bisphenol A (BPA), as well as BPS and BPF, because these industrial chemicals used in plastics and aluminum cans can seep into our food, disrupting the endocrine system and mimicking the effects of estrogen on the body. A number of health concerns have been linked with BPA, including an increased risk of cancer, infertility, obesity, and cardiovascular problems. It also has the ability to impact the brain, particularly in infants.

Unfortunately, avoiding plastics with the recycling codes #3 or #7 is nowhere near enough. That's because many products made with plastics that have been labeled BPA-free still contain other chemicals that can mimic estrogen. If you think about it, we use plastic for just about everything, simply because it makes life easier. We wrap our food up with it, heat our food in it, drink our water out of it, feed our babies from it, store our beauty products in it… You get the point. Replace your plastics with glass wherever possible, as this will provide your immune system with a little more protection from these toxic chemicals.

Hopefully most of us got the memo about our immediate need to toss out all cookware coated in non-stick coatings that contain the man-made chemical perfluorooctanoic acid (PFOA), which, incidentally, has been found to be present in most people's blood. I wish it was only present in this type of coating, as that would make getting rid of it far easier. Unfortunately, it has turned up in local water supplies, disposable coffee cups, stain-resistant carpeting, clothing, and flooring. Studies on animals have shown that exposure to PFOA increases the risk of tumors and cancer (including bladder cancer), and causes immune-cell change. To keep unwanted chemicals out of your foods, use non-toxic cookware coated with a ceramic non-stick layer.

Air filters and water purifiers

Air quality is highly influential when it comes to our health, and this is another area where we need to aggressively seek to keep toxins out of the body by removing them from our homes. Environmental toxins including tobacco smoke, air pollution, natural gas, and building materials in the home (such as carpeting, insulation, oil-based paints and stains, products made from engineered wood and plaster (which may contain asbestos), carcinogens, pesticides, formaldehyde, PFOA, polybrominated diphenyl ethers (PBDEs) and more) are endocrine disruptors. This means they are known to alter our hormone levels due to their toxicity, and therefore our exposure to them needs to be minimal.

Since we cannot control the air outside, we need to make sure we are controlling it inside our homes and offices as best we can. Toxin exposure can be dangerous to our health even in small quantities, increasing the risk of allergies and asthma, as well as liver, thyroid, and lung cancer. Air purifiers can remove more than ninety percent of airborne pollens, dust particles, virus particles, bacteria, pet dander, mold, and dust mites. HEPA filters purify the air by reducing air pollution in the home or office, providing you with cleaner air and reducing the toxic burden on your immune system.

I wish each one of us had the means to install a whole-house water filter system in our homes. Clean, filtered water removes carcinogens, sodium fluoride, and chemicals from our water. The hard water we are drinking, cooking with, and showering in contains excessive amounts of minerals, chlorine, chloramines, and heavy metals. Reducing chemical exposure is important for those with a compromised immune system, and filtered water supports overall health (especially seeing as we are primarily made up of water), which is one more strategy we can implement in order to alleviate environmental toxins.

If you cannot afford one for your entire house, you can get water filtration systems that go under the kitchen sink or, at the bare minimum, consider purchasing a water filter pitcher for your home. I recommend ZeroWater, which is the only filter pitcher to deionize the water and is comparable to the reverse osmosis system.

Exercise

As you begin to reduce the inflammation in your bladder and take your life back, it's important that you begin to incorporate exercise into your daily routine. If your IC symptoms are severe your common sense, coupled with your body's automatic response to the severity of the pain, will be to reduce mobilization to a bare minimum. The mere thought of exercise may seem daunting from where you are standing at this particular moment, but allow me to explain.

Exercise is multifaceted, in that it will strengthen your muscles, get your blood circulating and your heart pounding, stimulate the release of endorphins, increase energy levels, improve symptoms of depression, strengthen the immune system, relieve stress, and burn calories. Endorphins are neurotransmitters in the brain that are released during exercise, and this chemical release reduces our perception of pain, leading to feelings of euphoria. Since no two people are exactly alike, the level of endorphins released during exercise will vary from person to person, but I found that as long as the pain was not severe the high endorphin levels I got from exercise resulted in an almost immediate decrease in IC pain.

However, there is a line that you should be careful not to cross. Overdoing your exercise routine will almost certainly result in extreme pain later in the evening and in the days that follow. Like everything else we have discussed, begin slowly and use wisdom. Start with the goal of walking one block each day for the first week and build slowly from there, allowing your muscles time to adjust to the movement.

Pilates has truly transformed my body because it focuses on strengthening the core muscles and pelvic floor. I started with a Pilates DVD, beginning with the warm-up and then skipping ahead to the floor sequence portion. I opted for the easier modifications each time until

I developed enough strength to handle the entire workout without it irritating my bladder. My favorite Pilates DVD is *Element: Pilates Weight Loss for Beginners*, which I picked up for $10 at Walmart (and is also available at amazon.com).

If you suffer from diagnosed pelvic floor dysfunction (PFD), please disregard this section as you will need to work with a physical therapist and follow specified exercise guidelines. If you do not have a physical therapist or cannot afford one, you may experience positive results at home using a DVD called *Your Pace Yoga: Relieving Pelvic Pain*, which you can purchase at yourpaceyoga.com.

Pelvic floor dysfunction

According to statistics, 85% of woman with IC have pelvic floor dysfunction. This is an issue that affected me for some time before I realized what it was. As well as having the ability to cause leakage, PFD can cause pelvic pain. This impacted me separately from the usual bladder pain, particularly during times of stress.

The pelvic floor is the muscle group attached to the pelvic bone and scrum, supporting the rectum, uterus or prostate, and bladder, and wrapping around the urethra, rectum, and vagina. The way these muscles contract and relax controls our bladder and bowel functions, as well as affecting sexual function for women.

PFD can be caused by muscles that are either too tense or too relaxed. Those with IC who also suffer from PFD tend to have a combination of muscles that are too relaxed and too tense, so that they are effectively working against each other, which can cause the muscles to spasm. Symptoms may include frequent, urgent or painful urination; incomplete voiding or mid-flow stopping and starting; constipation or painful bowel movements; lower back, pelvic, genital or rectal pain; and pain during or after sex, or after sexual stimulation.

Pelvic floor physical therapy is proven to help in relaxing and desensitizing the central nervous system, which may help to ease symptoms in both the short and long term. Trained physical therapists may focus on posture, mobilization of joints and soft tissue, nerve retraining, muscle relaxation techniques, deep tissue massage, and myofascial release. They may also provide education on bowel or bladder-related issues.

Once again, the key to success is to look at the body as a whole, trying to understand the root cause of the problem and how one issue, such as

PFD, may affect another, such as IC, rather than treating these conditions in isolation. If any of these symptoms sound familiar, it may be worth asking your healthcare provider for a PFD physical therapy referral.

Essential oils

Essential oils are attracting a lot of attention these days. Everywhere I turn, someone I know is either talking to me about the benefits of using them or trying to sell them to me. I'll admit that I have been quite the skeptic! I don't believe that inhaling a "stress relief" essential oil will suddenly cause all anxiety to just melt away. I believe that wellness is integrated and comprises a range of functions. Therefore, we should pursue all avenues, taking a comprehensive approach to dealing with our overall health. Relying on essential oils as a be-all and end-all is simply not enough, especially when you take the functioning of essential pathways into consideration. However, when used in conjunction with everything else laid out in this book they can be extremely beneficial, and will add one more tool to your tool belt.

Essential oils are plant-based medicines that have been around for centuries and are used for both physical and emotional wellness. They are safe and effective when used correctly, but you need to be careful when selecting a brand. Not all are created equal, so make sure you select pure, organic, high-quality oils. They can either be inhaled, ingested, or applied topically, and knowing how to use each oil properly is extremely important. Make sure you read the instructions carefully to prevent unwanted side effects.

The top three essential oils are:

1. **Lavender**, which can be used directly on the skin for rashes, burns, wounds, and bug bites. It is also very calming, helping to relieve anxiety and stress. I rub it on the bottom of my feet at night if I'm having trouble sleeping.
2. **Frankincense**, which is calming, anti-inflammatory, and helps with skin issues. You can use it with an oil diffuser or massage it into the skin.
3. **Lemon oil**, which can help with mood, candida, infections (as it has antiseptic qualities), and lymphatic drainage. Diffuse five drops, or to boost your immune system mix two drops with half a teaspoon of coconut oil and massage into the neck.

Sauna

Finally, if you have access to a sauna and, more specifically, to a far-infrared sauna, regular usage will help you further rid your body of toxins, including heavy metal toxins. The skin is the body's largest organ, and sauna usage causes the skin to sweat, which aids detoxification. Toxins are stored in our fat as well as in our deep tissue, and can be eliminated from the body by means of perspiration.

According to the Global Healing Center, the use of saunas increases red cell and plasma volumes, strengthens the immune system (thus decreasing our chances of developing a cold), and aids in the detoxification of toxins stored within our fat and deep tissue. It also improves circulation and increases oxygen levels. The importance of eliminating toxins from the body cannot be overlooked, and therefore every avenue that may assist in detoxifying the body should be carefully considered.

Recommended supplements

Make sure you consult with your healthcare practitioner before using any of the following. Certain medications may interact with supplements, and some individuals may not be able to tolerate them. Also, seek to find balance here. Don't overload your system with vitamins, which can put too much strain on your system. Add one at a time, as needed, and once you begin to feel better rotate them and then seek to reduce usage. Below is merely a list of options, and it is not recommended nor advised that you take them all simultaneously. Once you feel more balanced you will only need to support areas in which you know you are prone to struggle.

General use supplements

All in One Multi-Vitamin/Mineral capsules from Holistic Health (holisticheal.com). This is the only multivitamin I know of that is bladder-friendly.
Hydroxy B12 Mega drops or Methyl B12 Mega Drops from Holistic Health (holisticheal.com) or Methyl B12 5000 MCG (store.amymyersmd.com).
Tryglyceride Omega-3 fish oil from SuperiOmega (amazon.com).
Liver Support (amymyersmd.com).

Bladder support

Cysto Renew Bladder Support from Douglas Laboratories (douglaslabs.com).

Aloe Vera Supplements from Desert Harvest (amazon.com).
Histamine Scavenger from Professional Health Products
(clinicalnutritioncenters.com).
Organic D-mannose powder from Micro Ingredients (amazon.com).
Organic coconut water (planetorganic.com).
Corn silk tea (amazon.com).
Marshmallow root tea (amazon.com).

Detox
Clear Change 10 Day Program with UltraClear Plus pH: a metabolic
detoxification program (available through a Metagenics-approved
practitioner, via metagenics.com, and sometimes at amazon.com or
doctorschoice.org).
OptiCleanse GHI from Xymogen (ask your doctor).

Treating infections/pathogens
Black Seed Oil 650mg (pure, cold-pressed) from Heritage Store
(amazon.com).
Oil of Oregano from Health Thru Nutrition (amazon.com).
Grapefruit Seed Extract ParaMicrocidin 250 (amazon.com).

Repairing leaky gut
Acetyl-Glutathione from Dr. Amy Myers (store.amymyersmd.com).
N-Acetyl L-Cysteine (NAC) from Integrative Therapeutics (amazon.com).
IgG Protect from Ortho Molecular Products(orthomolecularproducts.com).
Digestive Enzyme from Dr. Axe (store.draxe.com).
Betaine & Pepsin digestive enzyme from Ortho Molecular
(amazon.com) or HCL (betaine with hydrochloride) by Dr. Amy Myers
(store.amymyersmd.com).
L-Glutamine Powder 5g from Thorne Research (amazon.com).
Organic Bone Broth Collagen Pure powder from Dr. Axe
(store.draxe.com) or an organic bone broth of your choice. Drink 1-3 cups
per day as tolerable.
Zinc 30 from Pure Encapsulations (amazon.com).
Collagen Peptides (hydrolyzed) from Sports Research (amazon.com).
Vitamin D3 10,000 IU from Pure Encapsulations (amazon.com).
Vitamin A + Carotenoids from Pure encapsulations (amazon.com).
SBO Probiotic from Dr. Axe (store.draxe.com).

DGL Licorice Root Extract 400 mg from Natural Factors (amazon.com).
Quercetin 500mg (amazon.com).
Slipper Elm Bark from Nature's Way (amazon.com).
Caprylic Acid from Pure Encapsulations (amazon.com).
GI Microb-X from Designs for Health (amazon.com).

Gut support
GI Repair Powder by Dr. Amy Myers (store.amymyersmd.com).
Intestinal Repair Complex from Nutra BioGenesis
(nutrabiogenesis.com/intestinal-repair-complex-d57097.html).
GI Revive powder from Designs for Health
(catalog.designsforhealth.com/GI-Revive-Powder).

SIBO
Microb-Clear by Dr. Amy Myers (store.amymyersmd.com).
Primal Earth Probiotic by Dr. Amy Myers (amymeyersmd.com).

Candida
Candida Combat (store.draxe.com).
Candifense by Dr. Amy Myers (amymyersmd.com).
Probiotic Capsules 100 Billion by Dr. Amy Myers (amymyersmd.com).
Coconut oil (topical use).

Stress and anxiety
Neurocalm magnesium powder (Magnesium L- Threonate) from
Dr. Amy Myers (store.amymeyersmd.com).
Kavinace from NeuroScience (accutrition.com).

Thyroid Support
Thyroid Support Iodoral IOD 12.5 from Optimox (amazon.com).
Adrenal Support Adreset for stress and low energy from Metagenics
(store.drhyman.com).
Thyroid Calming from Dr. Amy Myers (amymyersmd.com).

*

Due to the constant assault on our bodies via the environment and food,
the fight to decrease the toxic burden while simultaneously increasing

detoxification will not come about without an intentional approach. An article written by a group of Harvard researchers caught my attention recently when it announced that six million Americans are living with what is considered to be unsafe drinking water containing detectable levels of industrial chemicals. We are drowning ourselves in toxins, and though we cannot move to our own little islands where we are completely safe from all harm, both seen and unseen, we can gather the facts, weigh up our options, and choose wisely. We can change our course and set sail in a new direction.

As you move forward in taking back your life and regaining your health, remember that it is a journey and will not happen overnight. Leave no stone unturned in your quest to figure out the root causes of your IC. Tune in to your body and listen to what it is telling you. It's speaking to you daily, and you have the choice to either listen or ignore it and continue doing things the way you have always done them.

If you are facing IC head on, understand that you did not just wake up sick one day. You got to this place over a period of time, so allow yourself time to heal. Strive to do what you can to take proper care of your body, remembering to treat yourself with kindness, gentleness, and love. This may seem strange, but I assure you that shifting away from a negative attitude toward self and training your thoughts so you can give thanks in all seasons of life will change your outlook. An attitude of gratitude fosters love, which should be the foundation from which you build as you seek to nurture your body back to health. Of course, there are days when I am lazy and cut corners, but I try to live each day making better and healthier choices than I did the day before. If you fail one day, remember that tomorrow is a new day, and that it will grant you a fresh start.

Your number-one goal right now needs to be reducing inflammation by eliminating anything that causes or contributes to it in the body. Once inflammation is eliminated and your body is balanced and calm, you can seek to prevent any further assault on your immune system by living an intentional life, whereby you refrain from causing it to become stressed out. Unfortunately, there is no quick fix for the majority of IC sufferers. Regaining your health will require change, and though you may be tempted to dig your feet in I want to encourage you to resist the urge to settle for just coping.

I have met many people who would much rather eat what they want whenever they want it, drink what they feel like whenever they feel like it, and live however they feel like living. They opt instead to take medicine, which allows them – usually only temporarily – to maintain the lifestyle they are accustomed to living. Very few will seek to get to the root of the issue and willingly change course with the intention of finding their healing by any means possible. Change is hard, but it's time for us to realize our own strength.

Plenty of people are living ordinary lives, but I want to live an extraordinary life! I have resolved that I will not step down from my quest until I have reached my desired goal, whatever it may be. If I was able to go from barely able to walk a block to being able to exercise daily; from a ridiculously strict diet to eating an entire grapefruit (a pleasure previously denied to me because of its citrus content); and from daily pain meds to no pain meds at all, I am certain that I can continue on this path, being ever mindful that each day is a gift. My immune system is strong once again, and I am able to kick a cold or virus in almost twenty-four hours. In fact, I made it through the entire winter season without catching a cold or getting the flu! Not only do I feel able and energetic, but I am in the best shape of my life, and the dietary restraints I once lived with are being lifted off more and more with each passing day.

The sweetest part is that I can now take care of my family the way I have always desired. And each night I get to curl up in bed next to the man I love the most; the man who has been my friend, my source of constant encouragement and my strongest supporter. Gone are the sleepless nights filled with pain, flare-ups, the constant need for a heating pad, the endless trips to the bathroom, and the glare of the T.V., which I previously lived by in order to distract myself. I have officially traded it all in for the dark peacefulness that surrounds me as I lie comfortably tucked into my bed.

Because there is an autoimmune component to IC, my journey with IC will never completely come to an end. I will always be prone to toxic overload and chronic inflammation. If I'm not careful, I know that the health of my gut could once again become compromised and that the health of my bladder could once again be affected. I also understand that specific pathways will need support in order to function. Therefore, I will live the rest of my life conscious of the fact that if I don't take care of myself my IC symptoms can, and most certainly will, come back. I will never take my health for granted again.

I wish I could hand you a single pill that would immediately cure all your problems, but unfortunately that's not the case with interstitial cystitis. If you want to send your IC into remission, or at least minimize your symptoms, you will have to do the work! However, I do want to encourage you in the fact that if I have been able to find my way back to health you can do the same thing! Choose to face this head on. Be strong, have faith, and don't give up until you have your life back. Each day I feel stronger and healthier, empowered by the knowledge and understanding that once eluded me, far more certain of the direction in which I am headed, and… alive! May you be encouraged to fight, determined to find answers, and resolved to finish your race.

IC Wellness
I am well aware that not everyone has access to alternative medical practitioners or integrative nutritionists. It is my heart's desire to help those who are seeking a heathier way of life as well as a community, so, in an effort to help those who wish to live healthy lives, I am in the process of establishing IC Wellness. This online resource will offer information, services, recipes, a store, a blog, and a patient forum, where you can connect with others within the IC community.

Please visit www.icwellness.org to find out more, and follow us on social media @ic_wellness.

FIVE-DAY MEAL PLAN
Day one

Breakfast (mango and banana smoothie)
Recipe by Elisabeth Yaotani

Ingredients
1 cup spinach
1 ½ cups coconut water
½ stalk celery
1 cup fresh mango
½ cucumber pealed
½ banana
1 scoop collagen powder
1 tsp spirulina (optional)
Directions
Place in blender, mix until smooth and enjoy!

Snack
Drizzle avocado with olive oil and sprinkle with Himalayan salt.

Lunch (vegetable salad)
Recipe by Elisabeth Yaotani

Ingredients
Organic Power Trio (spinach, kale, and chard)
Chopped carrots, broccoli florets, cauliflower florets, diced celery, sliced cucumber, and avocado
Apple cider vinegar
Olive oil
Directions
Mix all the vegetables together. Whisk 1 part apple cider vinegar with 3 parts olive oil. Add salt and pepper. Toss with salad mix.
Snack
Celery or carrots with organic hummus.

Dinner (pot roast)
Recipe by Lise Shadle

Ingredients
3.5 lb chuck roast
1 small yellow onion, sliced
2 cloves garlic
24 oz Yukon potatoes, cut in fourths
1 bay leaf
1 tsp avocado oil
½ tsp red wine vinegar
1 cup organic beef bone broth
1 tbsp sea salt (more to taste)
½ tsp pepper
Directions
Place meat in slow cooker and add all other ingredients. Cook on low for 8 hours. Serve with quinoa.

Day two

Breakfast (green apple smoothie)
Recipe by Elisabeth Yaotani

Ingredients
1 cup spinach
¼ cup broccoli
½ avocado
½ green apple
½ banana
1 cup frozen strawberries
1½ cups coconut milk
1 scoop collagen powder
Directions
Blend in blender until smooth.

Snack
Coconut yogurt with gluten-free granola.

Lunch (veggie omelet)
Recipe by Elisabeth Yaotani

Ingredients
3 eggs, beaten
1 tsp raw butter
Himalayan pink salt and pepper to taste
("Veggies") broccoli florets, green onion (finely chopped), and baby spinach
Cilantro, finely chopped
½ avocado, sliced
Sprouts
Directions
Melt butter in pan, add "veggies" and cilantro, then sauté for 4-5 minutes. Add eggs, then salt and pepper to taste. Cook on low until egg is cooked through. Top with avocado and sprouts.

Snack
Carrot and celery sticks with almond butter.

Dinner (chicken and spice)
Recipe by Elisabeth Yaotani

Main dish ingredients
2 organic chicken breasts
2 tsp sea salt
1 tsp cumin
1 tsp coriander
¼ tsp turmeric
½ tsp black pepper
1 tbsp avocado oil
Directions
Heat oven to 350 degrees. Line baking sheet with unbleached parchment paper. Mix seasoning (salt, cumin, coriander, turmeric, and pepper) in bowl. Coat chicken breasts with oil, then sprinkle seasoning on both sides of the chicken. Place chicken on lined baking sheet and bake for 12-15 minutes, depending on thickness of breast. Turn halfway through. Serve with steamed asparagus and sweet potato.

Sweet potato side dish ingredients
1 medium-sized, baked sweet potato
1 tbsp coconut oil
1 tsp cinnamon
½ tsp organic coconut palm sugar
Directions
Heat oven to 400 degrees. Line cookie sheet with unbleached parchment paper. Peel the skin from the sweet potato, rinse and dry with paper towel. Slice potato into ⅛-inch slices. Mix cinnamon and sugar together in bowl. Place potato slices on cookie sheet, lightly brush both sides with oil, then sprinkle with mixture. Bake for 20 minutes or until center is tender.

ELISABETH YAOTANI

Day three

Breakfast (real red smoothie)
Recipe by Brianne Gohlke

Ingredients
½ cup frozen beets, diced
1 cup frozen raspberries
1 cup seedless red grapes, stems removed
1 tsp fresh ginger, grated
1 cup water
1 tbsp ground flaxseed

Directions
Place all ingredients in a high-speed blender and mix well. Pour into a glass and enjoy!

Snack
Drizzle avocado with olive oil and Himalayan pink salt.

Lunch (veggie sushi rolls)
Recipe by Rose Manning

Ingredients
1 cup cooked sushi rice
4 toasted nori seaweed sheets
1 tbsp toasted sesame seeds, plus more for sprinkling
½ English cucumber, peeled and cut into thin matchsticks
½ ripe avocado, thinly sliced
4 romaine lettuce leaves
¼ cup water to seal the nori
Coconut aminos for dipping (optional)
Bamboo sushi mat

Directions
Place a bamboo sushi mat on the work surface with the bamboo strips facing you horizontally. Place the nori sheet horizontally, shiny-side down, on the mat, aligned with the edge nearest you. Spread the cooled rice over the nori sheet in an even layer, leaving the top ¼ of the nori uncovered. Sprinkle the sesame seeds over the rice, then arrange the cucumber and

romaine leaf and the avocado slices in a horizontal strip across the bottom portion of the rice.

Starting from the edge closest to you, lift the mat, nori, and rice over the filling to seal it inside, then roll the sushi into a tight cylinder. Use your finger to lightly moisten the outer edge of the nori with water to seal the roll. Dipping a sharp knife into the water before each cut, cut the roll in half crosswise, then cut each half crosswise into 4 equal pieces.

Pack the sushi snugly into an airtight container and sprinkle with sesame seeds. Refrigerate until ready to go. Include little containers of coconut aminos if you like to dip your sushi, and don't forget the chopsticks!

Snack
Seasonal fruit bowl. Cut fruit into bite-sized pieces and mix together. Sprinkle with Himalayan pink salt.

Dinner (salmon and capers)
Recipe by Elisabeth Yaotani

Ingredients
2 6oz fillets of wild-caught salmon
2 tbsp avocado oil
1 tbsp capers
1 tsp garlic, minced
1 tsp onion, minced
Sea salt and pepper to taste

Directions
Heat skillet over medium heat. Coat salmon in oil, garlic, and onion. Place in skillet and top with capers, salt, and pepper. Cook for three minutes, then turn and cook for another 3-5 minutes, or until it flakes easily with a fork. Serve with steamed broccoli and/or quinoa.

Day four

Breakfast (green breakfast bowl)
Recipe by Rose Manning

Ingredients
½ cup cooked organic brown rice
½ cup egg whites
½ cup broccoli
1 cup spinach
½ avocado
¼ cup fresh parsley
1 tbsp toasted pumpkin seed oil
1 tbsp toasted sesame seeds
2 tbsp avocado oil

Directions
Cook brown rice according to packaging instructions and set aside. Heat 1 tbsp avocado oil in a sauté pan. Add chopped broccoli and cook until almost soft, then add spinach and cook until slightly wilted. Place cooked broccoli and spinach in a bowl with your brown rice. Add 1 tbsp avocado oil , then add egg whites to the same sauté pan. Scramble until done, then place over the rice and veggies. Place sliced avocado next to the eggs, finishing with a drizzle of toasted pumpkin seed oil and a sprinkle of toasted sesame seeds.

Snack (smoothie)

Ingredients
½ cup coconut milk
½ cup pear juice
½ banana
handful of spinach
1 scoop collagen powder
½ cup ice

Directions
Place all ingredients in blender and mix until smooth.

Lunch (turnip, leek, and coconut soup)
Recipe by Rose Manning

Ingredients
1 large turnip, cut into chunks
1 leek, cut into strips
¼ cup watercress
1 can organic coconut milk (no sugar)
2 cups organic, no-salt or low-sodium chicken or vegetable stock (Imagine Broths are wonderful, but homemade is even better)
2 cups water
1 tbsp avocado oil
1 pinch Celtic sea salt
1 tbsp toasted pumpkin seed oil

Directions
Heat 1 tbsp avocado oil in a deep soup pan. Add leeks, and sauté until cooked through. Take out cooked leeks and set aside. In the same pan, bring 2 cups water to the boil and add the turnip. Cook turnip until soft and a fork passes right through.

Drain cooked turnips and place them back in the pot. Add your cooked leeks, watercress, coconut milk, broth, and Celtic sea salt. Blend all together, preferably with a hand blender. Once blended, reheat and serve with a drizzle of toasted pumpkin seed oil on top and more fresh watercress.

Snack
Air-popped popcorn sprinkled with Himalayan pink salt. (You could also add raw or imported butter if you are able to tolerate it.)

Dinner (grilled balsamic portobello "steak")
Recipe by Brianne Gohlke

Ingredients
4 portobello mushrooms
¼ cup balsamic vinegar or apple cider vinegar
Seasonings of choice (choose one or more from list below)*
2 garlic cloves

1 tbsp Dijon mustard
½ tsp ginger, grated
2 tbsp coconut aminos
1 tsp paprika
1 tsp dried thyme
½ tsp red pepper flakes

Directions

Remove stems from mushrooms and place gill side up on a baking sheet. Mix vinegar with your seasonings of choice. Spoon over mushrooms and marinate for a half hour. Preheat the grill to medium and grease with olive oil. Cook for 5 minutes, basting with vinegar mix after 2-3 minutes. Turn 90 degrees and cook for additional 3 minutes.

Flip to gill side down and cook for a further 3 minutes. Remove from grill and let it sit for 5 minutes before serving. Serve with steamed asparagus and baked sweet potato topped with imported butter and cinnamon.

Note: If you're using a countertop grill (i.e. George Foreman), learn from me and don't close the lid or you'll have an extra charbroiled Portobello!

* On my first round I only used vinegar to season; however, I would highly recommend garlic and mustard, or ginger and aminos, to give it some extra flavor.

Day five

Ingredients
½ cup oats (certified gluten-free, uncontaminated)*
1 ¼ cups unsweetened almond milk
½ tsp pure vanilla extract
¼ tsp cinnamon
1 tbsp ground flax seed
2 tbsp almond butter
1 banana, sliced

Directions
Add the oats, milk, vanilla extract, cinnamon, and flax seed to a jar or container, then stir. Refrigerate overnight (no longer than 3 days). On day of eating, heat if desired, then add banana and nut butter.

* Certified brands include: Bob's Red Mill, Cream Hill Estates, GF Harvest, Montana Gluten Free, and Avena Foods

Snack
Drizzle avocado with olive oil and Himalayan pink salt.

Lunch (pumpkin, chicken, and watercress salad)
Recipe by Rose Manning

Ingredients
Butterhead lettuce
½ cucumber peeled
½ cup fresh watercress
½ avocado
4 oz organic chicken breast
1 tbsp toasted pumpkin seed oil
1 tbsp toasted, unsalted pumpkin seeds
1 tbsp avocado oil

Directions

Heat avocado oil in a pan and add chicken breast. Once chicken is cooked through, set aside to cool. Chop butterhead lettuce, cucumber, watercress, and avocado. Place all your veggies on plate and top with cooked chicken breast, then finish with toasted pumpkin seed oil and a sprinkle of pumpkin seeds.

Snack (baked apples with cinnamon)

Core and chop 5 apples. Place in baking dish and bake at 350 degrees for 20 minutes. Remove from oven, then sprinkle with cinnamon and a handful of raisins.

Dinner (lentil soup)
Recipe by Naomi Synodinos

Ingredients

1 cup brown or green lentils
¼ cup onion, diced
2 cloves garlic, minced
1 carrot, diced
1 zucchini, diced
½ yellow bell pepper, diced
⅛ cup parsley, chopped
¼ cup avocado oil
¼ tsp cumin
1 tsp sea salt
4 cups chicken broth

Directions

Soak lentils for 12 to 24 hours beforehand, then rinse. Heat olive oil in pot and sauté onions, bell pepper, carrots, and garlic for 5 minutes. Add remaining ingredients, bring to the boil, cover, and reduce to simmer. Cook for 18–22 minutes. Add a splash of red wine vinegar 1 minute before it is done.

If soup is too thick, add broth or water to thin.

ELISABETH YAOTANI

WORKS CITED
AND FURTHER READING

Adams, M., "Vitamin B-12 warning: Avoid cyanocobalamin, take only methylcobalamin," Natural News, June 21, 2011: http://www.naturalnews.com/032766_cyanocobalamin_vitamin_B-12.html (accessed June 16, 2016).

Armstrong, L. "Lance Armstrong Quotes," BrainyQuote., 2016: https://www.brainyquote.com/authors/lance_armstrong (accessed March 12, 2016).

Aubrey, A., "Is Organic More Nutritious? New Study Adds to Evidence": http://www.npr.org/sections/thesalt/2016/02/18/467136329/is-organic-more-nutritious-new-study-adds-to-the-evidence (accessed March 23, 2017).

Axe, J., "7 Signs and Symptoms You Have Leaky Gut," n.d.: https://draxe.com/7-signs-symptoms-you-have-leaky-gut (accessed November 12, 2017).

Axe, J., "The Leaky Gut Diet and Treatment Plan", n.d.: https://draxe.com/leaky-gut-diet-treatment (accessed September 13, 2017).

Bazilian, W., *Eat Clean, Stay Clean* (New York: Rosdale, 2015).

Boldt, E., "9 Candida Symptoms & 3 Steps to Treat Them," Dr. Axe. March 2018: https://draxe.com/candida-symptoms (accessed January 11, 2018).

Bradstreet, A., "Ann Bradstreet Quotes," Goodreads, n.d.: https://www.goodreads.com/author/quotes/159922.Anne_Bradstreet (accessed May 26, 2016).

Brown, S. E. and Trivieri, L, Jr., *The Acid Alkaline Food Guide* (2nd edition, Garden City Park: Square One Publishers, 2013).

Carnahan, J., "Balancing Your Brian Chemistry: Treating Neurotransmitter Imbalances," Yakadanda, August 2011: http://www.jillcarnahan.com/2011/08/16/balancing-your-brain-chemistry-testing-and-treating-neurotransmitter-imbalances (accessed August 30, 2016).

Carnahan, J., "MTHFR Gene Mutation-What's the Big Deal about Methylation?", Yakadanda, May 2013: http://www.jillcarnahan. com/2013/05/12/mthfr-gene-mutation-whats-the-big-deal-about-methylation (accessed January 10, 2016).

Cousins, N., "Norman Cousins", BrainyQuote, n.d.: https://www. brainyquote.com/quotes/norman_cousins_121582 (accessed May 20, 2016).

Curtis, C. S. and Misner, S., "Pesticide Versus Organically Grown Food," The University of Arizona Cooperative Extension, Department of Natural Sciences, 2006: https://ag.arizona.edu/pubs/health/foodsafety/az1079. html (accessed September 29, 2016).

Davis, W., *Wheat Belly* (New York, NY: Rodale., 2011).

Detwiler, C., Mitchell, K., and Reichenbach, N., *Life by Design* (Boston: Cengage Learning, 2014).

Edison, T. "Thomas A. Edison Quotes", BrainyQuote, n.d.: https://www. brainyquote.com/quotes/thomas_a_edison_149049 (accessed April 26, 2015).

Finmore A., Roselli M., Britt S., Monsatra G., Ambra R., Turrni A., and Mengheri E., "Intestinal and peripheral immune response to MON810 maize ingestion in weaning and old mice," December 2008: https://www. ncbi.nlm.nih.gov/pubmed/19007233 (accessed June 10, 2017).

Forouzanfar, F., Bazzaz, B. S. F., and Hosseinzadeh, H., "Black cumin (Nigella sativa) and its constituent (thymoquinone): a review on antimicrobial effects," December 2014: https://www.ncbi.nlm.nih.gov/ pmc/articles/PMC4387228 (accessed April 2, 2017).

Forum user: "Question: Is there a simple explanation of the methylation cycle diagram?" Resqua.com, n.d.: http://resqua.com/100005927200207/ is-there-a-simple-explanation-of-the-methylation-cycle-diagram (accessed July 1, 2016).

Gandhi, M., "Mahatma Gandhi Quotes," BrainyQuote. n.d.: https://

www.brainyquote.com/quotes/mahatma_gandhi_122084 (accessed May 24, 2016).

Gardner, J. W., "John W. Gardner Quotes," BrainyQuote, n.d.: https://www.brainyquote.com/quotes/john_w_gardner_134413 (accessed April 1, 2016).

Gholipour, B., "What's in Urine? 3,000 Chemicals and Counting", TechMedia Network, September 5, 2013: http://www.livescience.com/39453-urine-chemical-composition.html (accessed May 23, 2016).

Gillies, T., "Society and superbugs: Losing 'one of the most serious infectious disease threats of our time,'" Thomson Reuters, October 2, 2016: http://www.cnbc.com/2016/10/02/society-and-superbugs-losing-one-of-the-most-serious-infections-disease-threats-of-our-time.html (accessed October 2, 2016).

Gohlke, B., "Diet Part Three: Let's focus on the details," February 2018: http://livinghealthylives.co/3232-2 (accessed March 5, 2018).

Green, P. and Jones, R., *Celiac Disease: A Hidden Epidemic* (New York, NY: HarperCollins, 2016).

Group, E., "5 Health Benefits of Sauna Use," February 2013: http://www.globalhealingcenter.com/natural-health/5-health-benefits-of-sauna-use (accessed September 20, 2016).

Jones, C., *Life is Tremendous* (Mechanicsburg, PA: Executive Books, 1968).

Kannall, E., "List of Nightshade Vegetables and Fruits," Livestrong, November 2, 2016: http://www.livestrong.com/article/534718-can-cayenne-pepper-hurt-your-stomach (accessed February 15, 2017).

Kresser, C., "RHR: Methylation 101," May 2015: https://chriskresser.com/methylation-101 (accessed February 3, 2018).

Levy, J., "The Most Common IBS Symptoms & What You Can Do About Them," April 2016: https://draxe.com/ibs-symptoms (accessed January 11, 2018).

Lynch, D. "MTHFR A1298C Mutation: Some Information on A1298C MTHFR Mutations," DBL Network, November 2011: http://mthfr.net/mthfr-a1298c-mutation-some-information-on-a1298c-mthfr-mutations/2011/11/30 (accessed July 02, 2016).

Malterre, T., "How Chemicals Increase Food Allergies and Sensitivities," Whole Life Nutrition, n.d.: https://www.wholelifenutrition.net/articles/food-allergies/how-chemicals-increase-food-allergies-and-sensitivities (accessed October 21, 2016).

Malterre, T., "Processed foods: How do they affect your body?" Whole Life Nutrition, n.d.: https://wholelifenutrition.net/articles/gluten-free/processed-foods-how-do-they-affect-your-body (accessed September 22, 2016).

McCoy, K., "Do You Have SIBO Symptoms? Here is All You Need to Know!" Dr. Axe, June 2018: https://draxe.com/sibo-symptoms (accessed January 08, 2018).

McIntosh, J., "What is serotonin and what does it do?" April 2016: https://www.medicalnewstoday.com/kc/serotonin-facts-232248 (accessed November 10, 2017).

Mercola, J., "Monsanto Decimates Their Credibility," September 2013, Dr. Mercola Premium Products: http://articles.mercola.com/sites/articles/archive/2013/09/10/monsanto-bt-corn.aspx (accessed July 12, 2017).

Mercola, J., "Women Put an Average of 168 Chemicals on Their Bodies Daily," Dr. Mercola Premium Products, May 2015: http://articles.mercola.com/sites/articles/archive/2015/05/13/toxic-chemicals-cosmetics.aspx (accessed October 28, 2016).

Miller, R., "Genetics 101: The Secrets Your DNA Holds," Tree of Life, n.d.: http://www.tolhealth.com/wp-content/themes/treeoflife-2017/pdf/dna-brochure-1805.pdf (accessed May 12, 2017).

Mohammadi, D., "Why bingeing on health foods won't boost your immune system," The Guardian, January 24, 2016: https://www.theguardian.

com/science/2016/jan/24/health-foods-immune-system-colds-vitamins (accessed June 13, 2016).

Monaco, E., "California Crops May Have Been Irrigated with Toxic Wastewater for 30 Years," Organic Authority, October 2016: http://www. organicauthority.com/california-crops-may-have-been-irrigated-with-toxic-wastewater-for-30-years (accessed November 3, 2016).

Moore, A., Aldington, J., Cole, P., and Wiffen, P.J., "Amitriptyline for neuropathic pain and fibromyalgia in adults," PubMed.gov, December 12, 2012: https://www.ncbi.nlm.nih.gov/pubmed/23235657 (accessed October 12, 2015).

Morrissette, D. A., "Psychiatric Disorders: A Messed Up MTHFR," Neuroscience Education Institute, n.d.: http://cdn.neiglobal.com/ content/blog/messed_up_mthfr.pdf (accessed July 10, 2016).

Myers, A., "The Problems with Grains and Legumes," Amy Myers M.D., April 2014: http://www.amymyersmd.com/2014/03/the-problem-with-grains-and-legumes (accessed May 24, 2017).

Myers, A., *The Autoimmune Solution* (New York, NY: HarperOne, 2015).

Myhill, S., "CFS - The Methylation Cycle," DoctorMyhill.co.uk, n.d.: http://www.drmyhill.co.uk/wiki/CFS_-_The_Methylation_Cycle (accessed December 27, 2014).

NewBeauty Editors, "How Toxic Are Your Beauty Products?" New Beauty, September 2014: https://www.newbeauty.com/video/972-how-toxic-are-your-beauty-products (accessed February 4, 2016).

Nickel, J. C., "Antibiotic Therapy for Interstitial Cystitis," National Institutes of Health, 2001: https://www.ncbi.nlm.nih.gov/pmc/articles/ PMC1476055 (accessed December 29, 2017).

Pick, M., "Digestion & GI Health – The Truth About pH Balance", Marcelle Pick OB/GYN, NP, April 2017: https://www.marcellepick.com/ digestion-gi-health-truth-ph-balance (accessed July 6, 2017).

Plagakis, S., "Amount of Toxics Released in the U.S. Increased for the Second Year in 2011," January 29, 2013: http://www.foreffectivegov.org/amount-of-toxics-released-increased-for-2nd-year (accessed November 3, 2016).

Rapaport, L., "Toxic chemicals in drinking water for six million Americans," Reuters, August 2016: https://www.yahoo.com/news/toxic-chemicals-drinking-water-six-million-americans-171010033.html (accessed October 16, 2016).

Roberts, J. C., "Approaches to Detoxification," EECP Center of Northwest Ohio, December 2014: http://www.heartfixer.com/CHC%20-%20Treatments%20-%20Overview%20Detox%20Options.htm (accessed July 1, 2016).

Robinson, C., Antoniou, M., and Fagan, J., *GMO Myths and Truths* (3rd edition, London: Earth Open Source, 2015).

Sant, G. R., Theoharides, T. C., Letourneau, R., and Gelfand, J., "Interstitial Cystitis and Bladder Mastocytosis in a Woman with Chronic Urticaria," ResearchGate, December 1996: https://www.researchgate.net/profile/Jeffrey_Gelfand/publication/13824548_Interstitial_Cystitis_and_Bladder_Mastocytosis_in_a_Woman_with_Chronic_Urticaria/links/5738a0bf08ae298602e2a417.pdf/download?version=va (accessed July 7, 2016).

Sant, G. R. and Theoharides, T. C., "The role of the mast cell in interstitial cystitis," National Institutes of Health, February 1994: https://www.ncbi.nlm.nih.gov/pubmed/8284844 (accessed January 3, 2018).

Smith, J., "Health Risks," Institute for Responsible Technology, n.d.: https://responsibletechnology.org/gmo-education/health-risks (accessed September 29, 2016).

Staff writer, "50 Jaw-droppingly Toxic Food Ingredients & Artificial Additives to Avoid," Public Health Analysis, n.d.: http://mphprogramslist.com/50-jawdroppingly-toxic-food-additives-to-avoid (accessed August 27, 2016).

Staff writer, "About NTP," National Toxicology Program U.S. Department of Health and Human Services, September 2016: http://ntp.niehs.nih. gov/about/index.html (accessed November 3, 2016).

Staff writer, "Amino Acids Analysis, Urine," Genova Diagnostics, 2016.: https://www.gdx.net/product/amino-acids-analysis-nutritional-test-urine (accessed September 21, 2016).

Staff writer, "Atarax," Drugs.com, December 2013: https://www.drugs. com/search.php?searchterm=Atarax&a=1 (accessed October 15, 2015).

Staff writer, "Big Question: Can your environment change your DNA?" *Duke Magazine*, August 2012: http://dukemagazine.duke.edu/article/big-question-can-your-environment-change-your-dna (accessed August 10, 2016).

Staff writer, "Cancer and Toxic Chemicals," Physicians for Social Responsibility, n.d.: http://www.psr.org/environment-and-health /confronting-toxics/cancer-and-toxic-chemicals.html (accessed November 3, 2016).

Staff writer, "Clear Change 10 Day Program with UltraClear Plus pH," Metagenics, n.d.: https://www.metagenics.com/clear-change-10-day-program-with-ultraclear-plus-ph (accessed January 17, 2018).

Staff writer, "How Thermography Works," Silk Thermal Imaging, n.d.: http://silkthermalimaging.com/how-thermography-works (accessed February 23, 2016).

Staff writer, "Interstitial Cystitis," Mayo Clinic, n.d.: http://www. mayoclinic.org/diseases-conditions/interstitial-cystitis/home/ovc-20251830 (accessed May 23, 2016).

Staff writer, "MTHFR Gene Mutation Explained," Glutathionepro Pro, n.d.: http://glutathionepro.com/mthfr-gene-mutation-explained (accessed January 6, 2016).

Staff writer, "Parabens in Shampoo – 5 Important Facts," n.d.: http:// sulfatefreeshampoos.org/parabens-in-shampoo-5-important-things-know (accessed October 10, 2016).

Staff writer, "Pesticide-Induced Diseases: Cancer", n.d., Beyond Pesticides:

https://www.beyondpesticides.org/resources/pesticide-induced-diseases-database/cancer (accessed September 29, 2016).

Staff writer, "The Best Way to Boost Your Immune System," Consumer Reports, December 2015: https://www.yahoo.com/news/best-way-boost-immune-system-185341589.html?ref=gs (accessed July 2, 2016).

Staff writer, "The Good, The Bad, and the Ugly," MastCellAware, n.d.: http://www.mastcellaware.com/mast-cells/about-mast-cells.html (accessed December 29, 2017).

Staff writer, "The Overuse of Antibiotics in Food Animals Threatens Public Health", ConsumersUnion, n.d.: http://consumersunion.org/news/the-overuse-of-antibiotics-in-food-animals-threatens-public-health-2 (accessed January 22, 2018).

Staff writer, "The Six Thousand Hidden Dangers of Processed Foods (and what to choose instead)," Body Ecology, n.d.: http://bodyecology.com/articles/hidden_dangers_of_processed_foods.php (accessed September 21, 2016).

Staff writer, "What is Interstitial Cystitis (IC)?" Interstitial Cystitis Association, January 2015: http://www.ichelp.org/about-ic/what-is-interstitial-cystitis (accessed May 23, 2016).

Staff writer, "What Is Interstitial Cystitis/Bladder Pain Syndrome?" Urology Care Foundation, n.d.: http://www.urologyhealth.org/urologic-conditions/interstitial-cystitis (accessed May 23, 2016).

Staff writer, "What is Oxalate?" Low Oxalate Diet Info, n.d.: http://www.lowoxalate.info (accessed January 24, 2017).

Staff writer, "What's wrong with modern wheat," GrainStorm Heritage Baking, 2016. https://www.grainstorm.com/pages/modern-wheat (accessed September 21, 2016).

Staff writer, "Wheat Flour," Pesticide Action Network, n.d.: http://whatsonmyfood.org/food.jsp?food=WF (accessed March 7, 2017).

Stengler, M., *The Natural Physician's Healing Therapies* (Stamford, CT: Bottom Line Books, 2013).

Stewart, K., "Methyaltion Overview for Professionals," NeuroSensory Centers of America, n.d.: http://www.drkendalstewart.com/wp-content/uploads/2011/09/Methylation-Overview-for-Professionals-10.11.pdf (accessed June 11, 2016).

Van Hoesen, S., "EWG's 2016 Dirty Dozen List of Pesticides on Produce: Strawberries Most Contaminated, Apples Drop to Second" December 2016: https://www.ewg.org/release/ewg-s-2016-dirty-dozen-list-pesticides-produce-strawberries-most-contaminated-apples-drop (accessed September 30, 2016).

Walia, A., "New Study Finds Roundup Herbicide to be 125X More Toxic Than Regulators Claim," Collective Evolution, April 2014: http://www.collective-evolution.com/2014/04/17/new-study-finds-roundup-herbicide-to-be-125x-more-toxic-than-regulators-claim (accessed April 6, 2017).

Walia, A., "Scientists Can Predict Your Pesticide Exposure Based On How Much Organic Produce You Eat," Collective Evolution, February 2015: http://www.collective-evolution.com/2015/02/23/scientists-can-predict-your-pesticide-exposure-based-on-how-much-organic-produce-you-eat (accessed April 5, 2017).

Whiteman, H., "1 in 2 People Will Develop Cancer in Their Lifetime," Medical News Today, February 2015: https://www.medicalnewstoday.com (accessed February 12, 2016).

Willis, A. K., *Solving the Interstitial Cystitis Puzzle* (Beverly Hills, CA: Holistic Life Enterprises, 2001-2003).

Wilson, D., "Understanding the Methylation Cycle and its Effect on Health," Dr. Doni, March 2015: https://doctordoni.com/2015/03/understanding-the-methylation-cycle-and-its-effect-on-health (accessed August 17, 2015).

Wilson, L., "Methylation," L. D. Wilson Consultants, April 2015: http://

drlwilson.com/Articles/methylation.htm (accessed July 11, 2016).

Wright, J. and Larsen, L., *Eating Clean for Dummies* (Hoboken, NJ: Wiley, 2011).

Yasko, A., *Feel Good Nutrigenomics Your Roadmap to Health* (Bethel, Maine: Neurological Research Institute, 2015).

Yasko, A., *Genetic ByPass Using Nutrition to Bypass Genetic Mutations* (Matrix Development Publishing, 2005).

Yasko, A., *Methylation Pathway Analysis* (Bethel, ME: Neurological Research Institute, 2015).

Yasko, A., "The Methylation Cycle," Dr. Amy Yasko, n.d.: http://www.dramyyasko.com/our-unique-approach/methylation-cycle (accessed June 7, 2016).

ELISABETH YAOTANI

INDEX